An Ibero-American Perspective on Narratives of Pandemics

ECOCRITICAL THEORY AND PRACTICE

Series Editor: Douglas A. Vakoch, METI

Advisory Board

Ecocritical Theory and Practice highlights innovative scholarship at the interface of literary/cultural studies and the environment, seeking to foster an ongoing dialogue between academics and environmental activists.

Recent Titles

An Ibero-American Perspective on Narratives of Pandemics

Edited by Zélia M. Bora, Animesh Roy, and Ricardo de la Fuente Ballesteros

LEXINGTON BOOKS
Lanham • Boulder • New York • London

Published by Lexington Books
An imprint of The Rowman & Littlefield Publishing Group, Inc.
4501 Forbes Boulevard, Suite 200, Lanham, Maryland 20706
www.rowman.com

86-90 Paul Street, London EC2A 4NE

British Library Cataloguing in Publication Information Available

Library of Congress Cataloging-in-Publication Data Available

ISBN: 978-1-7936-5404-5 (cloth)
ISBN: 978-1-7936-5405-2 (electronic)

Dedication
In memory of Anani Dzidzienyo, a Brown University
professor and connoisseur of Ibero-American culture.

Contents

Acknowledgments

This book is intended for those who are curious to explore the interrelationship between pandemic, environment, and literature in the Ibero-American region, particularly in Latin America. First and foremost, we would like to express our sincere gratitude to those who have supported and encouraged us throughout the creation of the book. Their belief and passion for this book project has been the key force behind its completion.

We would also like to extend our thanks to our contributors for working on such intriguing and complex issues and without whom the book would not have been possible at all. It is our sincere belief that this book will bring as much joy and inspiration to all as it has brought us.

We acknowledge our deep gratefulness to our editor Courtney Morales, and special thanks to Lexington Books, who worked tirelessly to bring the book to publication.

Finally, to our families who had to face all the inconveniences during the process of the book creation and who provided unwavering love and support throughout the writing process. Their patience and sacrifice allowed us the time, confidence, and the peace of mind to bring this book to life.

Thank you,
Zélia M. Bora
Animesh Roy
Ricardo Ballesteros de la Fuente

Preface

Zélia M. Bora, Animesh Roy, and Ricardo de la Fuente Ballesteros

The COVID-19 pandemic has had a profound impact on our lives including the ways we understand and engage with the environment around us. As we continue to grapple with the severe socio-political and economic consequences of the pandemic, it has forced us to reconsider the interrelationship between pandemic and environment, and address issues such as public health and environmental sustainability. This book is an attempt to look into the experiences of pandemics in select Ibero-American regions and how these experiences have been represented through literature and culture.

Ibero-American literature with its history of a rich social and political commentary has long explored the relationship between humanity and the natural world. Latin American literature in particular represents a deep attachment to the relationship between nature and identity, thereby playing a significant role in shaping national identities in the region. What is unique is that they all have used their craft to shed light on the complex issues the world is facing today. The sudden outbreak of COVID-19 and the experiences of the people in the Ibero-American region with the contagion has shifted the attention of readers to look beyond humanism and to examine the role of literature and culture in shaping public perception and understanding of pandemics and environmental issues. Ibero-American literature with its rich tradition of storytelling and cultural expressions provides a valuable lens to explore these issues and their impact on the individual and the community.

This book thereby tries to understand pandemics and to explore the ways such outbreaks are related to the larger environmental degradation and how Ibero-American literature and culture have tried to explore this interrelationship by questioning the impact of human actions on the environment.

It further tries to look into the cultural context of Ibero-America, the lived experiences of people during the pandemic, and how the culture has shaped the way pandemic and environmental issues are represented. By doing so, this book hopes to offer new insights not only into the pressing need to address the larger problems of the Anthropocene from a transdisciplinary perspective but also how literature can help us to make sense of the world in which we live.

Introduction

Narratives of Pandemic: Literature, Culture, and Environment—An Ibero-American Perspective

Zélia M. Bora, Animesh Roy, and
Ricardo de la Fuente Ballesteros

Much has been written about pandemics according to different fields of knowledge. However, there is still much to discuss in humanities, particularly the intriguing question about what it is to live in a post-pandemic world. The constant outbreaks of various viral diseases such as AIDS, Ebola, Zika, Monkeypox, and COVID-19 have left a feeling of deep health insecurity. Global access to air travel and other means of transportation has often proved to be conducive in the global transmission of viruses. In many ways, the world we lived in prior to COVID-19 doesn't seem like it will return. COVID-19 has affected societies and individuals around the world in more ways than we could ever imagine. Economically, individuals who were socially vulnerable were the most affected. Capitalism once again made the rich richer (see, e.g., Kelly 2020) and the poor poorer behind the curtain. Contemporary debates on pandemics as "natural" events have generally depoliticized pandemic responses, often obscuring the role humans play in creating pathways for transmission through the destruction of ecology. It is therefore essential to understand the triumvirate of ecological destruction, global warming, and pandemics.

Exploring the relationship between modernity and pandemics, historian Dipesh Chakrabarty, in his essay, "The Chronopolitics of the Anthropocene: The Pandemic and Our Sense of Time," demonstrates how the emergence of modernity and its development through industrialization, commercial manufacture of chemistry products, cars, refrigerators, aerosols, and inert gases have accelerated the process of global warming. Human consumption and

1

global increase of world population have overwhelmed the natural capacity of the planet to sustain itself. This crisis reached its climax in 2020 when the World Health Organization declared COVID-19 as a global pandemic (March 11, 2020).

Chakrabarty goes on to argue that "the pandemic and the climate crisis are connected phenomena. One could say that they both speak of Anthropocene times" (2021, 325). Chakrabarty also emphasizes that the Anthropocene "produces a peculiar sense of historical time." Defined as chronopolitics, the Anthropocene "plays out on different scales of time and space, both human and non-human" (Chakrabarty 2021, 326). In fact, the human role in the Anthropocene will be better evaluated through narratives that demonstrate how this crisis seems to be irreversible to future generations, if global efforts were not undertaken by the political leaders to ameliorate such a situation. The environmental crisis is also associated with neoliberal capitalism, a crisis of the industrial and consumption-oriented ways of human life. It is also a crisis of biodiversity, leading to what the scientists often refer to as the sixth mass extinction of species, or as a story of how humans fended off the next ice age by many thousands of years (Chakrabarty 2021, 326).

Such a tragic destiny that haunts the future of humans and non-humans alike has become a current phenomenon due to zoonotic exchanges between humans and non-humans. These facts have led experts to affirm that we now live in an era of pandemics, newly emerging infectious diseases, and the return of old contagious foes.[1] It is also clear that though science has a very precise idea about pathogens and infectious diseases as basic causes of pandemics, it however often remains focused on a few diseases and in the process other illnesses such as tuberculosis and mental disorders like melancholy, apathy, and depression are often ignored and have silently reached the status of global pandemics. Such diseases have reached epidemic proportion and most importantly they have increased particularly during modernity. These diseases have affected thousands of youngsters who died of consumption while others completed suicide in Europe and the Americas. The basic fact assumptions here are: 1) all the experiences (both literary and non-literary) are related to modernity; 2) all of them tell narratives of the Anthropocene related to illnesses of early modernity in Spain and Brazil and late modernity in Brazil, México, Guatemala, and Ecuador; 3) epidemics and pandemics are events that express the crisis of modernity as well the paradoxes of neoliberal economic model; and 4) memory and recollection are important processes to retrieve and understand the relationship between pandemics and environmental crises.

With better understanding of viral and bacterial diseases and their relationship to environmental destruction, this book calls for the need to historicize pandemics in light of their social and cultural realities. Our perspective also emphasizes aesthetic texts related to tuberculosis, apathy, and madness in the nineteenth century and the first decade of the twentieth century. The rest of the chapters are miscellaneous writings on COVID-19 in countries like Mexico, Guatemala, Brazil, and Ecuador.

MEMORY OF PANDEMICS: LIVING THE CONCEPTION OF A "BEAUTIFUL DEATH"

Various incidents have left a permanent scar on the twentieth-century consciousness and collective memory. Among them "examples of totalitarian barbarity, genocides comprising slavery, colonial exploitation and abject complicity in the American and European dictatorships in both West and East. It also includes political and military violence, economic disasters, health crises and intimate horrors of sexual violence" (Brian, Jaisson, and Mukherjee 2011). As health crises, epidemics and pandemics have countless narratives as part of humanity's collective memories that have survived through oral and written accounts and also through objects and places that represent human endurance, spirit, and resistance against illness. First written through medical chronicles, these narratives were also written by poets who have undergone the loss of their beloved relatives and friends. Their narratives symbolically represent the memory of thousands and various untold stories.

Literary narratives on Western plagues were first popularized through medical reports and historical chronicles. Pioneering the first literary narrative on plague in the West, Renaissance writers such as Boccaccio, Dante, Petrarch, and Chaucer brought to light the narrative of the first global pandemic, the Black Plague (see Farrell 2020; Ha 2021). Interestingly, in such literary narratives, accessory themes such as sexual drive of the characters was in sharp contrast to the constant presence of death in real life. The explicit sexualized conduct of the characters represents symbolic "spaces of freedom" that only imagination could achieve. Therefore, eroticism stabilizes the levels of reality, by indicating what is real and not real. Unlike real people, characters in the text are free and can transpose the limitations of time and morality and fear of contracting diseases.

During the late medieval period, death "surprised" the world in an unbridled and unstoppable race promoted by driven capitalism (see, e.g., Welsenthal and Alloway 2021). Trade and industry developed in thirteenth-century Italy, favored because of its trade routes (Welsenthal and Alloway 2021). As a result, death became a fatal event that put an end to feudalism and strengthened capitalism. Narrators were sometimes witnesses to and at the same time victims of the plague. Boccaccio witnessed some of his relatives and acquaintances die. Writing, in this case, represents the collective experience of the community the writer was part of. Though these narrators were often socially privileged, they did not necessarily belong to the dominant political group who controlled the politics of capitalism specially the exploitation of nature, as well as humans. Contrary to these privileged narrators, peasants and lower classes were impacted hard during pandemics. Historians have argued "that this labor shortage allowed the survivor peasants demanding better pay or seek employment elsewhere. Despite government resistance, serfdom and the feudal system itself were ultimately eroded" (Russel and Parker 2020).

The sense of narrating the collective experience represented through the literary texts during Romanticism did not have the same vitality of the Renaissance's texts regarding eroticism and the general concept of "good death." Instead, the idea of dead eroticism and disillusionment added a melancholic feeling and a tone of permanent loss. It was the time of the *mal du siècle*. By the end of eighteenth century in Europe, tuberculosis began its fatal outbreak. It was consumption that stereotyped the popular idea of the romantic poet who died young. The survivors were left with feelings of disillusion, apathy, melancholy, and depression. At that time, these diseases were understood as mental conditions defined as *mal du siècle*.

In the chapter titled "Tuberculosis Vaccine Development: Its History and Future Directions," tuberculosis is described as an ancient plague and a bacterial disease that has survived over seventy thousand years and that has affected nearly two billion people worldwide. It was first "noticed" during the Middle Ages when bubonic plague became an agent of severe contagion and death. It persisted during the Industrial Revolution and persists even today (MacDonald and Izzo 2015). During medieval times, it was known by the name of scrofula. In England and France, it became known as "king's evil" (Barberis et al. 2017). In their essay, Krugman and Chorba (2022) argue:

Many religious traditions have had thaumaturgic (relating to supernatural powers) touch as a tradition. In Britain, reference to the monarch as having divine power in "the royal touch" dates to the 11th century, when it was believed that Edward the Confessor, last of the Anglo-Saxon kings, possessed powers to heal the sick through some form of laying on of hands. In official ceremonies in his and subsequent reigns, subjects could approach the monarch to seek the imperial touch, hoping to cure their ailments or diseases. For centuries, the disease that most readily lent itself to the occasional appearance of success in this regard was scrofula (i.e., lymphadenitis—most commonly tuberculous cervical lymphadenitis), which would manifest itself with painful and visible sores that could go into remission and even go into resolution, giving the impression of a royally induced cure.

In the nineteenth century with the fading away of the "monarch's divine powers," other forms of rationalizing the illness were established. The disease affected artists, royals, and the impoverished population. It was considered variously as the white plague, the white death, or the wasting disease. In the chapter, "Morality, Mortality and Romanticizing Death Consumptive Chic: A History of Beauty Fashion and Disease," the interrelationship between consumption and fatal death gave rise to an attitude of resignation based upon evangelical principles as well as a cultural conception based on the notion of a 'beautiful death' (Day 2017, 41).

In this volume, chapter 1, "Tuberculosis and Melancholy in the Work of Gustavo Adolfo Bécquer" by Juan Pascual Gay and Mercedes Pascual Zavala, explores how tuberculosis influenced the notion of a "beautiful death" in Spain:

> it was represented as a sort of unattainable love since a death sentence weighed over the beloved. The inaccessibility thrived in the supposed purity of the beloved woman, until consumption was transformed into a synonym of beauty. The symptoms proper of tuberculosis (interior burning or bodily consumption) were similar to the experience of falling in love, so a correspondence between the feeling and the illness was settled. Romanticism formulates tuberculosis as an expression of love, conceived as the illness of passion.

Gay and Zavala also observe how such a concept became one of the most predominant characteristics of the Romantic aesthetics. The feeling of being mentally ill had a direct influence particularly reflected in the work of Gustavo Adolfo Bécquer. Considered as a "mystery and acutely enough feared will be felt to be morally, if not literally contagious" (Sontag 1978, 4), the disease was also connected to melancholy. Regarding melancholy, Bécquer refers to melancholic state as inseparable from tuberculosis as a cause of the spleen that possesses him (Gay and Zevala, this volume). Lacking essential material resources, Bécquer succumbed to a fatal death. His experience with modernity reached its limits in a fleeting world he did not have time to enjoy. Through his poems, he creates one of the most dramatic images that ever existed in the romantic context: the image of a young intellectual struggling to minimize the effects of a disease he knew was fatal. One can imagine how he dedicated his last days to his beloved work while some time was left. But unfortunately, there was no such a time left to him. Perhaps this fatal vision was particularly emphasized by the end of nineteenth century when the "infection rates in some cities were thought by public health officials to be nearly 100%. TB was also considered to be a sign of poverty or an inevitable outcome of the process of industrial civilization. About 40% of the working-class deaths in the cities were from tuberculosis" (Harvard Library n.d.). To sum it up, the memory one has from this collective affliction is that the concept of "beautiful death" was an attempt to come to terms with the inevitable and hopeless disease that would take the individual through a painful death. To the Romantic generation, wishing a beautiful death was after all a sort of self-appeasement of redeeming life that was finally and inevitably ending.

APATHY, MELANCHOLY, AND MADNESS: CRITICAL SCRUTINY AND BEYOND

In Greek culture, the word "apathy" was related to stoic philosophy; in the contemporary medical context, it is described as a debilitating syndrome associated with neurological disorders (Le Heron, Apps, and Husain 2018). Nonetheless, certain issues related to apathy, melancholy, and madness need to be emphasized by looking into these issues beyond the nineteenth-century approaches and by exploring the realities of the social subjects involved who were affected by the disease. According to Ricardo de la Fuente Ballesteros and Juan R. Coca in "The Turn of the Century and the Spanish Imaginary Facing the Disease: The Case of Ganivet" (this volume), the Basque poet Ángel Ganivet based his own experiences with apathy and melancholy, and discussed the term in a broader context identifying the illness both in personal and collective terms. However, as Ballesteros and Coca stress, Ganivet failed to correlate the social implications of the disease. At the time the poet lived, Spain in particular was facing a huge crisis because of mass immigration, agrarian crisis, social and religious conflicts, as well as political revolutions.

Nonetheless, in terms of ideas, the word "apathy" acquired more complex meanings, especially under the scientific ideas based on Darwin, Spenser, Nordau, and Lombroso. In the nineteenth century, the word "apathy" was considered as a sort of "mental degeneration." The word degeneration "came to be an umbrella term which seemed to give coherence to many elements of *fin de siècle* culture" (Clear et al. n.d.). "It was regularly invoked by contemporary commentators as the cause of the supposed increases in recidivistic criminal behavior, homosexuality, insanity, prostitution and poverty" (Barberis et al. 2017). Outside the European continent, particularly in Latin America, the reception of these ideas had serious implications on the social and racial policies regarding the nation formations. Allied to these ideas, the economic determination and the "natural" stratification of European society, according to capitalist establishment, long excluded since the seventeenth century and further marginalized most of the social contingent. As demonstrated by Foucault in his classic *Madness and Civilization*, this population were composed of the poor, unemployed, prisoners, and the insane (Foucault 1988, 39). Foucault's remarkable work on madness demonstrates how the European idea of confinement of "the dangerous classes" was an attempt to adequate generations of marginalized population after the end of feudalism to the new economic necessities and the pedagogy of capitalism. By linking the power of the ruling class and their association with the upbringing pedagogy of capitalism, people were confined. However, the failure of the Houses of Confinement was proved to be an ineffectual remedy to the nascent industrialization (Foucault 1988, 55), while mendicancy and idleness were considered as sources of all disorder, and "sloth became the absolute form of rebellion, the idle would be forced to work, in the endless leisure of a labor without utility or profit" (Foucault 1988, 57).

By alluding to the relationship between idleness and madness Foucault states that,

> it was in these places of doomed and despised idleness, in that space invented by a society which had derived an ethical transcendence from the law of work, that madness would appear and soon expand until it had annexed them. The nineteenth century would consent, would even insist that to the mad and to them alone be transferred these lands on which, a hundred and fifty years before, men had sought to pen the poor, the vagabond, the unemployed. (Foucault 1988, 57)

As Foucault exemplifies, the madman would be characterized by his inability to work and to follow the rhythms of collective life (Foucault 1988, 58). Regarding the origins of poverty, it was not related to the scarcity of commodities or unemployment, but "the weakening of discipline and the relaxation of morals" (Foucault 1988, 59). The Houses of Confinement, of which the Hôpital Général was one, "had the power of a moral, judicial apparatus and means of repression: 'they had the power of authority, of direction, of administration, of commerce, of police, of jurisdiction, of correction a punishment'; and to accomplish this task 'stakes, irons, prisons, and dungeons' were put at their disposal'" (Foucault 1988, 59).

To sum up, the House of Confinement in the Classical Age constituted the symbol of that "police" which conceived of itself as the civil equivalent of religion for the edification of a perfect society (Foucault 1988, 63). Until the end of eighteenth century, the Age of Reason confined demented men and individuals of wandering mind and persons who had become completely mad (Foucault 1988, 65).

The social impact of madness as part of the degeneration concept in the Americas followed, more or less, the European pedagogy and experience. In the case of Brazil, the first House of Confinement, besides the prisons, was Hospício D. Pedro II.[2] According to Marco Filho (2014), this mental institution was constructed following the best architectural design during the Brazilian empire, and it was inaugurated on July 8, 1841.Characterized as a

Panopticon, the building was constructed according to the philosophical and juridical proposal of Jeremy Bentham, to be a prison:

> Se baseou na vigilância do paciente, do estudante, do operário, ou presidiário e pressupunha a existência de mecanismos disciplinadores e normatizadores. No caso do Hospício de D. Pedro II, sua construção era em forma de anel, apresentando um pátio interno e, ao centro uma torre com vigia. (Filho 2014)

> It was based on the surveillance of the patient, student, worker, the prisoner and presupposed the existence of disciplining and regulating mechanisms. In the case of the D. Pedro II Mental Institution, its construction was in the form of a ring, with an internal courtyard and, in the center, a tower with a lookout. (Filho 2014)

Few years after the foundation of D. Pedro II institution, it became overcrowded and therefore had to face several problems regarding the administrative services:

> A decadência do Hospício foi refletida pela percepção da sociedade de que os objetivos propostos pela medicina não atendiam as demandas em relação à crescente população que ameaçava a organização da cidade. Os recursos diminuíam na mesma proporção em que a demanda aumentava e o Hospício perdia sua função terapêutica. (Filho 2014)

> The decline of the Hospice was reflected by society's perception that the objectives proposed by medicine did not meet the demands in relation to the growing population that threatened the organization of the city. Resources decreased in the same proportion as demand increased and the Hospice lost its therapeutic function (Filho 2014)

The general acceptance of individuals institutionalized regardless of their social status exemplifies the state of a "social" pandemic atmosphere characterized by madness. As it is suggested, mental disorders will amplify as long as the social demands become more severe to individuals who "fail" to fulfill those social and professional requirements. The impact of social Darwinism in Brazil created obstacles to the nation. The realization that Brazil was a "mixed-race nation" created new dilemmas for Brazilian social scientists (Schwarcz 2003, 165):

> Misto de cientistas e políticos pesquisadores e literatos, esses intelectuais se moveram nos incômodos limites que os modelos lhes deixaram, haja vista que, naquele momento, indagar sobre que nação era essa significativa, de alguma maneira, se sobre raça era a nossa ou então se a mestiçagem tão extremada não seria um sinal em si de decadência e enfraquecimento. (Schwarcz 2003, 168)

The mix of scientists, politicians, researchers, and literati moved within the uncomfortable limits of these models which were left to them. To question these limits were very significant to them. In some ways, they asked how race was an important category to the nation or if miscegenation was not a sign of decadence and weakening of the nation.

The *fin-de-siècle* in Brazil was lived with great pessimism. Some intellectuals were disillusioned with the promise of equality and tried to understand the persistent cause of differences among humans. Most of them were adept in polygenist theories of analysis. They understood race as an essential and ontological phenomenon resulting from the creation. These intellectuals concluded that "the evolution found in nature was exactly same as that expected for human beings. They supposed that the inferior groups constituted barriers to the progress of civilization" (Schwarcz 2003, 169).

One of the intellectuals who resisted the influence of social Darwinism to explain the degeneration of poor Black and brown communities was Lima Barreto. He demonstrated through his innumerous newspaper articles, short stories, and novels the social injustices perpetrated against the poor classes harassed by racism and political abandonment. In the chapter "The Language of a Sick Nation: Epidemics and Environmental Destruction in the Narratives of Lima Barreto," Zélia M. Bora explores the relationship between epidemics in the First Republic, social marginalization, and environmental destruction. It also highlights how social Darwinism influenced interregional racism in Brazil. The belief in racial hierarchy contributed to the social exclusion of these communities or their descendants in general. In a metaphorical sense, degeneration represented a "biological disease" that prevented the social mobility of most of the individuals that belonged to these groups. Finally, Bora, by exploring the moral disease of its main character, analyzes the meanings of madness in Lima Barreto's novel *Triste Fim of Policarpo Quaresma*. In her reading, immorality defines the madness of the novel's main character. Lima Barreto suggests how Brazil, in his time, was a sick nation not only because of the proliferations of epidemics that succeeded one another but also due to the immorality of their politicians.

WHEN VIOLENCE, DEATH, AND DISEASE BECOME A MEMORY THAT RESISTS DISAPPEARING

In places such as Guatemala, the gloomy atmosphere of death due to COVID-19 brought back emotions of intense loss among the indigenous Mayan population due to the loss of their cultural group during 1981 to 1983, particularly in the Ixil region.[3] Variously regarded as the Silent Holocaust or the Guatemalan Genocide, the incident was fatal for the entire Mayan population due to the fact that women, children, and the elderly were the ones to fall victim to what many consider one of the most violent phases in Guatemalan history. In this volume's chapter titled "Guatemalan Expressions: Memorials and Private Reflective Spaces during the Internal Conflict and COVID-19 Pandemic," Martha C. Galván-Mandujano demonstrates how the mnemonic process and educative work succeeded as strategies to recover and remember the past as well as to educate the community against COVID-19. Galván-Mandujano suggests how the spirit of resilience of a community is the outcome of a continuous effort. After the civil war, the Mayan community focused again on the ancestral struggle of their land, and the process of healing was intensified through the use of murals by the communities that kept the memory of the dead alive. Trying to historicize the context, Galván-Mandujano argues:

> The agrarian conflicts were happening and continued during the pandemic. According to PBI in Guatemala, in April 2020 in the worse part of the pandemic, families denounced publicly that they were being forced to evacuated, private entities (landowners and private companies) forced them. The government, and other international entities were not able to help. Washington, a community in Baja Verapaz conformed of 70 families, forced to work since the XIX century for landowners (finqueros) was evacuated. PBI Guatemala stated that "the families from the community of Washington lived now in the municipalities of Purhulá y Salamá with family members and friends. Now that they have been evacuated, they have difficulties surviving, since their crops were ubicated in the lands they lived was their means of subsistence."

Galván-Mandujano suggests not only the permanent of the indigenous people for the land but also the social and environmental catastrophe provoked by the abandonment of their lands. Galván-Mandujano goes on to argue that:

> During the pandemic many Achí Mayans were affected again economically due to travel restrictions bringing memories of struggle from the internal conflict. Since they could not go to Guatemala City because of government mandates. They relied in aid from organizations such as ADIVIMA and CONAVIGUA. In 2020 and 2021, these NGOs provided food assistance with the international help of organizations such as Trócaire, an agency of the Irish Catholic Church.
>   In general, genocide memorials serve multiple purposes. These include honoring the memory of victims, serving as symbolic forms of reparations, acting as sites of healing, bearing witness, and aiding in truth and justice initiatives. In the case of recent COVID-19 deaths, many cemeteries have been assigned only for these deaths. I broadly define memorials to include monuments, murals from the internal conflict, murals for COVID-19 awareness and honoring, cemeteries, spaces for COVID-19 deaths in cemeteries, and private reflective spaces associated with remembrance, memorialization and to teach about the pandemics.

The relevance of Galván-Mandujano's chapter relies first in demonstrating how monuments and murals are important elements in the process of communication between the indigenous population and the outsiders. The process includes learning, remembering, and healing as basic steps to restore individuals and collective identities in communities. In addition, it provides the reader a contemporary account of the ancient struggle for the land and the hardships in this contemporary survival.

INDIGENEITY, SYMBOLIC INSURGENCIES, POLITICAL SPIRITUALITIES, AND HEALING

Another significant chapter related to COVID-19 and its association with the indigenous experiences is written by María Fernanda Solórzano Granada. In her chapter "Between Life and Death: Practices of Healing of the Ecuadorian Siona Nationality as a Political Spirituality," Granada explores how in Ecuador and Colombia, the Siona People like all indigenous nationalities have a profound cultural attachment to the land. Most of Granada's chapter deals with the indigenous practices using herbs for the religious purpose of healing and protection. Together with *ujas* (healing songs), Granada considers the use of herbs as a form of cultural resistance. Granada uses terms such as "symbolic insurgences" and "political spirituality" to characterize the use of sacred plants, like *yagé* (ayahuasca) and *yocó* (*paullinia yoco*) that are used to heal spiritual and physical illnesses. Granada aims to show how the Siona people faced COVID-19, taking into consideration their cultural knowledge on herbs and how they collated it with the knowledge of their ancestors. By doing so, the Siona people symbolically restored their living contact with nature. Together, their knowledge of herbs symbolically brings the wisdom of their ancestors. According to Walsh (2013) and Granada,

> The nature/environment as a way of healing for indigenous communities represent their feelings, thoughts and practices into their cosmos and within an insurgent territory that allows them to constitute themselves as a collective political subjectivity; that is, as political subjects in the face of developmental and extractivist processes. For this reason, the sacred plants ceremony and their medicinal plants, has more than a simple vision of the world, it is a way to re-existence and resistance. (Granada, this volume)

THE CHALLENGES TO "NORMAL LIFE" AFTER PANDEMIC

Another problem in the lives of the rural population in Mexico during the pandemic was their geographical and economic isolation after the spread of COVID-19. Like other communities, the information depended on outsider sources, such as an effective process of communication by the government, non-governmental organizations, and the internet particularly for the reopening of schools at the elementary level. Norma Georgina Gutiérrez Serrano's chapter, "Now That We Are Back to School . . . Pandemic, Environment, and Community Links," describes the community of Benito Juarez Elementary School in San André de la Cal, municipality of Tepozclan, Morelos, and delves into how important the reopening the school was to the community.

The community is characterized by the defense of their territory and their way of life and reproduction. This ranges from the epic revolutionary battles of *Zapatismo* at the beginning of the twentieth century to more recent struggles against large-scale governmental and global projects such as plans to build golf courses, open up new highways, and put in chairlifts that would require cutting into the Sierra del Tepozteco hillside, as well as development projects that would directly affect aquifers and the fragile system of rainfed crops, directly destroying the habitat of local flora and fauna. The project would also alter the mythical ancestral landscape that has sheltered the Tlahuica and mestizo cultures of the region for centuries. The strength of these community ties is rooted in ancestral ways of working the land, and life in the community underlies the defense of their land, their customs, and the culture of the region. There is a deep sense of caring for the environment, all with profoundly vital community ties, as some authors describe (Martinez-Salazar 2014; Velasquez 2022; Haraway 2016; as well as Serrano, this volume).

Despite the historical tradition of the communities, return to school activities after one year and four months of class suspension meant the community had to face several challenges. It is also important to emphasize the community ties and efforts of cooperation among the residents and former residents (who work temporarily in the crops in the United States and Canada). This rural community inhabit a forest region where land use is based on ancient communal use and traditions. Most of them are engaged in agricultural works. Regarding the spread of COVID-19, it is suggested that the disease reached the community from their migrant members who brought the disease with them from the United States or Canada even though, according to Serrano, the community had one of the lowest rates of contagion. As Serrano argues, this is a type of education that takes place in community spaces, where sustainable productive practices are preserved and ways of life closely linked to cultural traditions are maintained, all the while simultaneously interacting with contemporary urban culture. Perhaps for these reasons, and because of everyday life outdoors, it recorded the lowest Covid indices in the country.

By using a self-ethnographic method, Serrano uses students' oral accounts, written compositions, drawings, and life stories where experiences and relationships are interrelated. Serrano's narrative gives the reader a sense of proximity and interaction within this specific society to understand how important it is to comprehend the indigenous ultimate plea for protection and salvation of nature. Historical records prove that plagues and illnesses have been reaching the indigenous communities in the Americas for centuries. Political and physical violence for the possession of their lands is complementary to this tragic reality. Incidentally, the struggle for the preservation of their land is also the struggle for the preservation of the planet. They are the last guardians of nature and the planet. Without them, all the life in the planet would be wiped out.

HOW TO THINK OF PANDEMICS, AND WHAT IS ITS RELATIONSHIP WITH THE ECOSYSTEM?

Georgina Vega Fregoso explores the question of the interrelationship between pandemic and environment in her chapter "Chronicle of Life during the COVID-19 Pandemic in Mexico"; from three different perspectives—researcher, mother, and housewife—Fregoso enables the reader to understand the interrelationship among different actors during the confinement. Among these actors, she considers her children, neighbors, and the inhabitants of a rural community. This methodology allowed her to contrast their fears, values, beliefs, and expectations about the risk of contracting COVID-19 with her own feelings. Based on these elements, she also considered the presupposition that the "imaginaries and subjectivity of social actors are constructed during the pandemic in their relationship with the environment and health" (Castoriadis 2005). Fregoso also adds important information on the history of Mexican epidemics and its social impact on poor population.

By emphasizing the "contemporary" incidents of the COVID-19 pandemic, she emphasizes the permanent state of transmission of different virus such was the case of influenza, a H1N1. She argues that:

> This approach, which emphasizes that deaths from COVID-19 have been much smore than those reported by the Secretary of Health in Mexico, has been

recovered by some national mass media through their journalists who are certainly not epidemiologists, experts in biostatistics or health professionals. On the other side are the downward perspectives, which consider that there were not or have been so many deaths caused only by the pandemic, but that the deaths can be attributed to other causes that are synergistic to the SARS CoV 2 virus, taking as a reference, in addition to the health records, other pre-existing clinical, environmental, social and economic variables.

Finally, she also analyzes the impact of the public efforts to fight the disease.

VULNERABLE COMMUNITIES AT RISK: BRIEF THOUGHTS ABOUT INDIGENOUS AND BLACK POPULATION IN BRAZIL

On May 19, 2020, World Vison International (2021) declared Brazil as the epicenter of the pandemic in Latin America, with 262,545 confirmed cases and 17,509 reported deaths—a figure that was just behind the United States and Russia. In Brazil, the Amazonian region was the most affected because of its demography and the heterogeneity of its population. The most economically vulnerable populations during the pandemic were the indigenous people and the Blacks, besides marginal communities such as riverside dwellers, inhabitants of favelas, and refugees. Historically, the indigenous and quilombola population in the Amazon has represented a high percentage of the entire population of Brazil, and their vulnerability is associated with the natural and socio-political challenges over their territory. "'Twelve of twenty states in the Amazon area had the highest incidence of cases of the disease and five out of ten municipalities were with highest mortality rate. Hospitals have run out of beds health workers are overwhelmed and there are horrific scenes of mass graves. This is making it difficult for families and even for funeral homes to provide quick and timely services,' said World Vision Brazil Response Director" (World Vision International 2021). One of the similarities between the indigenous and the Afro-Brazilian population in the Amazonian region was susceptibility to death due to their particular migratory demography, intensified by the outbreak of COVID-19. Both populations face on a daily basis pendular migration and return to their habitation due to their daily labor displacements, "in search for medical-hospital assistance and consolidation of political and legal visibility within the cities, where they regularly trans-migrate (Baines et alli 2013 3).

Due to the problem of access to information as well as the economic diversity of its population the daily routine of the inhabitants facilitated the social contagion.

Among the indigenous peoples of the savannah region in the Northeast of Roraima state on the border with Guyana and Venezuela, known locally as the *Lavrado* and *Serras* there are constant flows of people between the villages located on indigenous lands and the city of Boa Vista, the state capital, many of whom have residences on an indigenous land and in the city where they carry out work during part of the year. They commonly spend several months of the year working at their villages, and several months working in Boa Vista, in different jobs, but predominantly as construction workers in the case of men, and domestic servants in the case of women. Those who work in regular jobs in Boa Vista as public servants, in health services, teachers, and a few lawyers and other professionals usually live permanently in the city, but these constitute a small minority (Baines at all 2021 3).

Milanez in his paper, "Fighting the Invisible Anaconda" points out how it is essential to understand the relationship between virus resistance and the increased number of victims within indigenous (specially in this case the *Mura* people) and black population. Milanez argues that the problem "has been acting as a reactive signal to mark the numerous critical challenges involved in achieving the ways of life of native peoples" (Milanez 2020). Besides, the common problems that afflict the population, Brazilian ethnic and environmental racism is based on forging the various "other insiders" of the nation (Pacheco 2006).

The region has a history of endemic and chronic diseases such as dengue, yellow fever, smallpox and others as well as "the violence of contact relations with the populations of the cities and the pressing threat of hunger caused by the predation of forest resources were menacing the reproduction of traditional Amazonian territories, now, as a result of the pandemic, we stand before a clear threat to the physical, and cultural existence of several of the segments that inhabit the region" (Baines at all 2021). The confluence between the two groups take place mostly during the fishing season in the river Tiriaçu that has its course arranged in the western region of the state of Maranhão.

The complexity that surrounds the geographic areas also include movements between indigenous lands in Roraima, the capital Boa Vista, and the region of Guyana close to the Brazilian border:

Indigenous people depend on spending periods in their residences in their villages and access to communal Indigenous lands to produce horticultural products for their own family consumption, as well as selling any excess locally to obtain small amounts of money to buy basic manufactured goods. They also depend on spending periods in their residences in the capital of Roraima, Boa Vista and return regularly to their villages and periods spent in the city has been going on over several decades. (Baines, de Castro Pereira, and dos Santos 2021, 8)

Such details underline the basic problems faced by the indigenous and Black population who live in the Amazonian region. The geographical location, social isolation, and systematic racism prevent them from having better access to health and education. As a result, they have to migrate to urban locations on a daily basis to work on civil construction sites (men) and as domestic services (women), thus facilitating the transmission of the virus. The COVID-19 pandemic victimized mostly elders in these communities. The loss of elders endangered their cultural tradition. There is also the physical violence perpetrated by landowners and exploitation due to illegal mining and land occupation. It is not a coincidence that, over the last four years, loosening of government public policies regarding the protection of indigenous lands has intensified deforestation. Eco-fascism in association with climate denial and the destruction of human and non-human subjects are two complementary agendas. Therefore, the expectation related to a more egalitarian society appears impractical. Bringing these assumptions into the pandemic and post-pandemic context, Brazilian socio-political realities cannot be generalized to a political agenda that often ignores the deep social and historical inequalities inherent within. Regarding the pandemic and Amazonian territory, which represents well Brazilian paradoxes, the indigenous peoples are the last guardians of the forest. Once they abandon the forest, deforestation will continue until the last tree has been felled.

REVISITING TERMS SUCH AS NECROPOLITICS AND GENOCIDE UNDER COVID-19

In the chapter "Afro-Brazilian and COVID-19: Revisiting the Concepts of Necropolitics and Genocide," Siddharth Singh Monteiro Bora and Evely Vânia Libanori try to locate and reconsider necropolitics and genocide in the Afro-Brazilian context. Although the chapter deals specifically with Afro-Brazilian insertion in the context of COVID-19, it sees Blackness as a symbolic condition not only determined by socio-historical background but also capitalism and postcolonialism that has transformed otherness into a perpetual circle of dispossession that millions of individuals are subjected to. This study is once more a reflection on the experiences of representation in which meta-texts such as color, poverty, brutality, sexual license, and death are the products of necropolitics. Genocide and necropolitics are complementary strategies implemented by the formal state socially and economically over segregated populations. It can be intentional, rapid, and continuous like the death camps institutionalized by the Third Reich, and also in the native land of the subjects as in the case of Guatemala, during the establishment of authoritarian military regimes or by neglecting the populations and denying the basic services, as was the case during the COVID-19 pandemic.

VIRTUAL MEDIA AND COVID-19:
A LINGUISTIC APPROACH

The deadly dance of death of COVID-19 that has cost the lives of millions in countries like the United States and Brazil was politicized in the form of a war unleashed at the level of communication. The battlefield was the internet, and the method to reach the "passive" internet user was social media. In the chapter "Language and Pandemics: Uses and Effects of WhatsApp—Students and Teachers under Isolation," Juarez Nogueira Lins selects a particular context and considers the role of textual genres. These linguistic motivators are essential to understand some of the dynamics related to the intercommunication among users in order to evaluate how the dissemination of fake news and threats worked on a social marked context. In this case, WhatsApp was the virtual platform of analysis while the sample survey was done on university students and professors. Some of the conclusions that L. A. Marcuschi reached were "the impact of digital technologies on contemporary life has enormous power both to build and to devastate." Thus, "in this bias, the genres of the digital sphere, an unlimited source of interaction, by virtue of their reach and strength, can become 'weapons' in the hands of the unscrupulous, with the purpose of manipulating, deceiving, attacking interactants taking them at certain times, like in the case of the pandemic, to moments of euphoria, fear, sadness, aversion, depression" (Lins, this volume).

APPROACHES TO RE-THINK
ENVIRONMENTAL ETHICS

What are the lessons left behind by the pandemics? How can environmental ethics influence individuals to think about a better relationship with the environment in the post-pandemic world? These are the basic questions introduced in the last two chapters—"The COVID-19 Pandemic and Agency for a New Environmental Ethic" by Maria Geralda de Miranda and Bruno Matos de Farias, and "Biopolitics and the Environmental Governance in Time of the New Coronavirus Pandemic" by Marcus Alexandre Cavalcanti and Kátia Eilane Santos Avelar. In the former chapter, de Miranda and de Farias underline a particular set of ideas starting with Peter Singer's ethical perspective on environmental issues. The language of the text is objective and appropriated to the reader who is introduced to the issues for the first time. By introducing Latin American critics like Viveiros de Castro, the authors revisit classical philosophers as well as an indigenous perspective. In this amalgam of ideas, the most important is to question the role of the environment in our lives for the survival of the planet.

In the chapter "Biopolitics and the Environmental Governance in Time of the New Coronavirus Pandemic," Cavalcanti and Avelar emphasize sustainability as an essential pre-condition to minimize the effects of environmental degradation and therefore the inevitable spread of ancient virus and bacteria originating from flora and fauna. Based on the theoretical concepts of Foucault, Edgar Morin, Felix Guattari, and Enrique Left, the authors stress the complexity of the problem and its multiple perspectives that ranges mainly from socio-cultural to political dimensions. Although not emphasized in the chapter, the problems related to environmental devastation depend exclusively on the public policies implemented by the governments in each continent and nation. Politicizing the cause is the worst option to deny the relationship between pandemics and environmental degradation, and that is a slow passage from destruction to total chaos. Unfortunately, the existence of counter-narratives underlined by political denialism about global warming, pandemics, wars, famine, violence, and the constant harassment and death of the other are not considered outmost factors that will lead mankind to destruction. After all, we are dealing all the time with an incessant number of narratives, most of them degrading.

Even a cursory glance of this volume and the multiplicity of voices involved would lead us to understand the relationship between pandemic and environment and to accept that there are more questions than answers. Our world is increasingly being stressed each day by the scarcity of resources and the inability of the environment to respond to human needs; the human responsibility and influence over the acceleration of natural disaster is undeniable. There lies a huge gap between the combined public environmental policies of the North and the South with regard to the preservation of the environment, and only by merging this gap and addressing the root of the problem can we achieve a balance between nature and sustainable forms of development and any form of environmental justice.

NOTES

1. David Morens and Dr. Anthony Fauci, Director of the Institute of Allergy and Infectious Diseases (quoted in Chakrabarty 2021, 328).

2. Hospício de D. Pedro II da Construção à Desconstrução, http://www.ccms.saude .gov.br/hospicio/hospicio. See "A Superlotação: A Superlotação ," by Marco Antonio Moraes Filho, http://www.ccms.saude.gov.br/hospicio/superlotacao.php.

3. According to the Guatemalan Truth Commission, the army massacres destroyed 626 villages, and more than two hundred thousand people were killed or disappeared while 1.5 million were displaced by the violence and 150,000 were driven to seek refuge in México. The report by La Comisión para el Esclarecimento Histórico (CEH)—or Comission to the Historical Enlightment—found the state responsible for 93 percent of the acts of violence and the guerrillas (Guatemalan Revolutionary Union) responsible for the 3 percent. The victims were 83 percent Maya and 17 percent ladino. Victoria Sanfor demonstrates that 1) massacres were not the result of the rogue field commanders and 2) massacres were a systematic and strategic campaign of the army as an institution represented by General Rio Montt (1981–1982) and General Lucas Garcia (1982–1983.

REFERENCES

Barberis, I., N.L. Bragazzi, L. Galluzzo, and M. Martini. "The History of Tuberculosis: From the First Historical Records to the Isolation of Koch's Bacillus." *Journal of Preventive Medicine and Hygiene* 58, no. 1 (2017): E9–E12.

Baines, Stephen Grant, Márcia Leila de Castro Pereira, and Potyguara Alencar dos Santos. "Afro-Indigenous Cosmographies of Mobility: Fishes, Viruses and Others Amazonian Lives at the Confluence With the Sars-CoV-19." *Frontiers in Sociology* 5 (2021).

Brian, Eric, Marie Jaisson, and S. Romi Mukherjee. "Introduction: Social Memory and Hypermodernity." *International Social Science Journal* 62, no. 203/204 (2011): 7–18

Castoriadis, Cornelius. *A Instituição Imaginária da Sociedade Rio de Janeiro* 2 ed Paz e Terra 1982

Chakrabarty, Dipesh. "The Chronopolitics of the Anthropocene: The Pandemic and Our Sense of Time." *Contributions to Indian Sociology* 55, no. 3 (2021): 324–48.

Clear, Derek, Matt ffytche, Margaret Homberger, James Lister, and Tracey Loughran. n.d. "Introduction." *Deviance, Disorder, and the Self.* http://www7.bbk.ac.uk/deviance/intro.htm

Day, Carolyn A. "Morality, Mortality and Romanticizing Death." In *Consumptive Chic: A History of Beauty Fashion and Disease*, 41–52. London: Bloomsbury, 2017.

Farrell, Jenny. "Writing at A Time of Plague: Boccaccio, Dante, Petrarca, Chaucer." *People's World*, August 14, 2020. https://www.peoplesworld.org/article/writing-at-a-time-of-plague-boccaccio-dante-petrarca-chaucer/

Filho, Marco Antonio Moraes. "Hospício de Pedro II: da construção à desconstrução." 2014. http://www.ccms.saude.gov.br/hospicio/hospicio.php

Foucault, Michel. *Madness and Civilization: A History of Insanity in the Age of Reason.* NY: Vintage, 1984

Ha, Sha. "Plague and Literature in Western Europe. From Giovanni Boccaccio to Albert Camus." *International Journal of Comparative Literature and Translation Studies* 9, no. 3 (2021): 1.

Haraway, J. Donna. *Staying with the Trouble. Making Kin in the Chthulucene.* Durham, NC: Duke University Press, 2016.

Harvard Library. "Tuberculosis in Europe and North America, 1800–1922." n.d. https://curiosity.lib.harvard.edu/contagion/feature/tuberculosis-in-europe-and-north-america-1800-1922

Henry, Patrick. "Economic Inequality has Deepened during the Pandemic that Doesn't Mean It can be Fixed." *World Economic Forum*, April 7, 2020. https://www.weforum.org/agenda/2022/04/economic-inequality-wealth-gap-pandemic/

Le Heron, C., M.A.J. Apps, and M. Husain. "The Anatomy of Apathy: A Neurocognitive Framework for Amotivated Behaviour." *Neuropsychologia* 118 (2018): 54–67.

Kelly, Jack. "The Rich Are Getting Richer During the Pandemic." *Forbes*, July 22, 2020. https://www.weforum.org/agenda/2022/04/economic-inequality-wealth-gap-pandemic/.

Krugman, Jean, and Terence Chorba. "When a Touch of Gold was Used to Heal the King's Evil." *Emerg Infect Dis* 28, no. 3 (2022): 765–67.

MacDonald, Elizabeth M., and Angelo A. Izzo. "Tuberculosis Vaccine Development—Its History and Future Directions." In *Tuberculosis: Expanding Knowledge*, edited by Wellman Ribón. London: IntechOpen, 2015.

Mankikar, Kalpit. "China's Economy is Paying the Cost of Political Lysenkoism." *Rasina Debates*, May 16, 2022.

Martinez-Salazar, Egla. *Global Coloniality of Power in Guatemala: Racism, Genocide, Citzenship.* Lanham, MD: Lexington Books, 2014.

Milanez, Felipe. "Fighting the Invisible Anaconda Amidst a War of Conquest: Note of a Genocide." *Ambiente & Sociedade (Sicelo Br)*, São Paulo V.23 (2020).

Pacheco, Tania. "Inequality, Environmental Injustice, and Racism in Brazil: Beyond the question of Color." *Development in Practice* 18, no. 6 (2018).

Russel, Eleonor, and Martin Parker. "How the Black Death made the Richer, Richer." BBC Future. *Worklife*, 2020.

Sontag, Susan. *Illness as Metaphor and AIDS and Its Metaphor.* NY: Macmillan Picador, Farrar et al., 1978.

Schwarcz, Lilian Moritz. "O Espetáculo da Miscigenação." A Recepção do Darwinismo no Brasil. Domingues, Heloisa Maria Bertol et all coleção História e Saúde, 2003.

Velasquez, Teresa A. *Pachamama Politics: Campesino Water Defenders and the Anti-Mining Movement in Andean Ecuador.* Tucson: University of Arizona Press, 2022.

Walsh, Cahterine. *Pedagogias decoloniales: Practicas insurgente de resistir, (Re)existir y (re)vivir.* Tomo I Quito, Ecuador: Ediciones, Abya-Yala, 2013.

Welsenthal, Joe, and Tracy Alloway. "How the Black Death Pandemic Reshaped Europe's Feudal Economy." *Bloomberg*, January 9, 2021. https://www.bloomberg

.com/news/articles/2021-01-09/how-the-black-death-pandemic-reshaped-europe-s
-feudal-economy#xj4y7vzkg

World Vision International. "Our Response." 2021. https://www.wvi.org/emergencies
/coronavirus-health-crisis/our-response

PART I

Chapter One

Tuberculosis and Melancholy in the Work of Gustavo Adolfo Bécquer

Juan Pascual Gay and Mercedes Pascual Zavala

Tuberculosis (TB) is an illness readily associated with Romantic beauty. According to Isabelle Grellet and Caroline Kruse (1983), this Romantic motif appeared in England around the time of the Industrial Revolution. The prestige that Romanticism ascribed to fragility is taken on as a topic. Moreover, TB was soon regarded as the ailment of artists and writers, to the point where it became the *mal du siècle*, above even pessimism and *ennui*. TB drew the attention of romantic artists because for as long as its causes remained unknown it was a misunderstood affliction since it stood for the relentless loss of a life. The mysterious origins of the disease exacerbated imaginations.

It represented unattainable love, since a death sentence weighed over the beloved. The inaccessibility thrived in the supposed purity of the beloved woman, until TB was transformed into a synonym of beauty. From that moment on, TB and beauty operated as synonyms. The symptoms proper of TB (interior burning or bodily consumption) were similar to the experience of falling in love, so a correspondence between the feeling and the illness was settled. Romanticism formulates TB as an expression of love, conceived as the illness of passion. The disease's progression was proportional to the resignation. At the same time, patients with consumption were not expected to exist much longer and polluted their surroundings with pessimism, as a result of the loss of vitality. This explains the fact that, from Romanticism, the anemic state was projected toward natural environment to the point of becoming its contiguity. Nature was an extension of that this state, without a solution of continuity between the patient's sensibility and the outside.

25

Gustavo Adolfo Bécquer (1836–1870), a conspicuous figure of Spanish Romanticism, fell ill with consumption during 1857 and, after overcoming the first diagnosis, gravely relapsed in 1863. Consequently, he traveled to the Cistercian monastery of Veruela on that year, at the Moncayo's foot in the province of Zaragoza, accompanied by his brother Valeriano. During this period, he continued to collaborate with Madrid newspaper *El Contemporáneo* with a series of letters, which were later assembled under the title of *Desde mi celda*, included en *Obras completas* (1969).[1]

The importance of TB in Becquer's poetry and prose does not exclusively stem from the fact that he suffered from it, but also from an embedded metaphor capable of engendering further metaphors pertaining to sickness. Becquer speaks of consumption as a consumptive himself, but also as a writer, for he espouses a set of meanings, entrenched in the Romantic movement itself, that go beyond the individual's ailment. In this sense, Becquerian TB irrupts both explicitly and implicitly throughout his writing, to the point of becoming inseparable from it. Some rather clear instances of this are those pertaining to femininity and illness, but these are not the only symbols inseparable from consumption. Other such symbols are melancholy or ruins—occasionally related to the feminine, always subscribing to illness. Metaphors drawn from this larger metaphor that is TB enriches and gives cohesion to Bécquer's texts. TB does not operate exclusively as a literary topic but as a poetic principle. Sometimes, his oeuvre even strikes as being irreducible to the illness.

Throughout the century, consumption is qualified as a "sick flower" or as "venom hidden among the flowers." Melancholy is also closely related to this affliction. It seems as if black humor is the anemic equivalent of what consumption is in physiological terms. Klibansky, Panofsky, and Saxl indicate that "At the beginning of the nineteenth century, however, a type of melancholy arose out of this strange dualism of a tradition gone stale and the spontaneous and intensely personal utterance of profound individual sorrow—namely, the 'romantic' melancholy" (Klibansky, Panofsky, and Saxl 1979, 238). Romantic melancholy embraces reality in order to underline the splendor of what it exhibits through rich and profuse language. This attitude answers to the artist's pain, who explores the transience of beings and objects in order to appropriate beauty. Consumption provides the individual with both experiences. It resolves itself in a self-regarding search whereby melancholic pain turns toward the ephemeral nature of existence, which is in turn corroborated by the illness. It irrupts throughout the tragic Romantic poetry that preceded the decaying *Weltschmerz* in which, according to J.P. Jacobsen (1978, 237) "toda belleza es belleza que se desvanece" (all beauty is beauty that fades away).

This attraction toward the ephemeral as the definitive expression of beauty was already presented in Romanticism. Etymologically, TB embodies the meaning of the Spanish word "*tisis*," "consumption" or "deterioration of the organism." Miguel de Covarrubias, in his *Tesoro e la lengua castellana o española*, defines the "tisical" voice as "enfermedad mortal, que tiene su asiento en los pulmones, y los enfermos se van consumiendo y secando" (mortal disease that affects the lungs; Covarrubias 1998, 963). In *L'Encyclopedie* (1751), Diderot defines it as small tumors.

In *Illness as a Metaphor*, Susan Sontag adds something meaningful: "Tuberculous appeared as a prototype of passive death" (Sontag 1978, 40). The agent of pulmonary affection, Koch's bacillus, was discovered in 1882. Consumption was already the illness par excellence, defining the nineteenth century. The relationship between TB and the bourgeoisie has been stated on numerous occasions. But this distinctive aspect of the illness was rescinded when it became known that the disease was caused by unsanitary environments, to which the working classes were far more exposed. Cleared from its aristocratic patina, this finding relegated consumption as an artistic and literary concern.

During the final years of the nineteenth century, there are two predominant models of femininity: the "femme fatale," inseparable from the decadent movement, and the ethereal virgin associated with the pre-Raphaelites. The femme fatale is the result of the destructive decaying Weltschmerz. The pre-Raphaelite feminine is a herald of masculine annihilation, reactive to explicit illness, a result of its reaction against Victorian academicism. Dante Gabriel Rossetti in "Lilith from Gothe" presents the vampires:

Hold thou thy heart against her shining hair,
If, by thy fate, she spread it once for thee. (Rossetti 1911, 542)

For pre-Raphaelites, what remains from the Romantic feminine is its appearance. In Bécquer it is already introduced at the beginning of "La ajorca de oro." In *El pacto con la serpiente*, Mario Praz registers the characteristics of this proposal, related to the inflence of Poe, Baudelaire, and Wagner (Praz 1988, 111). But the pre-Raphaelite feminine ideal carries its sources on its sleeve. In some ways, it is a sophisticated and quintessential extremity of Romanticism. Salvador Dalí, in "Le surréalisme spectral de l'éternel féminin preraphaélite," foregrounds the tension between the pre-Rafaelite feminine and the end of the century's morbidity (Dalí 1936, 47). The pre-Raphaelite woman rejects the precise illness that is inseparable from romantic beauty, but not the melancholy that foreshadows morbid aspects of the *fin du siècle*. The cause of this gravity can be found in TB, as Sontag writes: "TB is a disease of time; it speeds up life, highlights it, spiritualizes it" (Sontag 1978, 14).

This mysticism seeps into to the pre-Raphaelite feminine, but is bereft from its pathological origin. In the tale "Un boceto natural," Bécquer introduces Julia as an elegant and delicate woman and, despite her ironic expression, she is innocent and mysterious (1969, 717).

> En aquel momento llegó Julia: parecía otra mujer; nada más ligero y elegante que su sencillo traje de color de rosa; nada más fresco y gracioso que su sombrero de paja de Italia, cuyas anchas cintas de oro blanco se anudaban debajo de su barba con un gran lazo de puntas sueltas y flotantes. Estaba descolorida, como el día anterior, pero sus facciones eran tan delicadas que la luz parecía transparentarse a través de ella. Sus inmensos ojos, cuyas pupilas se dilataban desmesuradamente en la misteriosa sombra del crepúsculo, estaban entonces entornados, como definiéndose de la deslumbradora claridad del día. En sus labios delgados y encendidos, en los cuales creí observar en mi primera entrevista una expresión irónica, brillaba una sonrisa tan ingenua e inocente como la de los niños cuando se ríen durmiendo, porque según sus madres ven pasar a los ángeles sobre su cabeza. (717)

> At that moment Julia arrived: she looked like another woman; nothing was more elegant and lighter than her simple pink suit, nothing fresher and more gracious than her hay hat from Italy, which's wide white-golden ribbons tied under her chin with a huge knot of loose and floaty ends. She was discolored, like the day before, but her features were so delicate that the light look transparent through her. Her immense eyes, which pupils dilated immeasurably in the mysterious shadow of twilight, were then half closed, as if defending herself from the dazzling clarity of the day. In her thin and lit libs, upon which I believed to see in my first interview an ironic expression, such ingenuous and innocent smile shone, like the children's when they laugh in their sleep, because according to their mothers they see the angels pass above their heads.

In similar ways, he describes the protagonist in "El beso" (1969, 282). He also emphasizes the pink tone of Sara's lips and her white dead complexion:

> Tenía los ojos grandes y rodeados de un sombrío cerco de pestañas negras, en cuyo fondo brillaba el punto de luz de su ardiente pupila como una estrella en el cielo de una noche oscura. Sus labios, encendidos y rojos, parecían recortados hábilmente de un paño de púrpura por las invisibles manos de un hada. Su tez era blanca, pálida y transparente como el alabastro de la estatua de un sepulcro. (1969, 293)

> In the pupils of her great eyes, shadowed by the cloudy arch of their black lashes, gleamed a point of light like a star in a darkened sky. Her glowing lips seemed to have been cut from a carmine weft by the invisible hands of a fairy. Her complexion was pale and transparent as the alabaster of a sepulchral statue.

The ephemeral and episodic characteristics are inevitably linked to the Romantic feminine. It all seems to suggest that the Romantic devotion for sickly beauty is tied to the interest in ruins, which will operate as a symbol for decay later. Ruins fascinate on two levels: they are both the vestige of a famous past and testament to the destructive power of nature. They are the result of an intrinsic disparity in terms of the experience of time. The consumptive woman also incarnates this experience but inverts its orientation: it is the appearance of threatened present before its imminent disappearance. The dichotomy between Classic and Romantic art established by Goethe, or the one drawn by Schiller between naive and sentimental poetry can here be felt as a reformulation of the old clash between ancients and moderns. Therefore, the first term of the dichotomy is characterized by vitality, the second one, by illness. To the Romantic eye, however, not even Greek Art could be spared from darkness (Colli 2020, 73). To Rafael Argullol, sickly beauty is linked to ruins, as they are both expressions of the Dionysian exhibition of drunkenness, morbidity, and subjectivity (Argullol 1987, 24). It denotes an array of paradoxical and contradictory senses. The epidemic of TB spread to the arts up to the point where it became a decisive motif of the Romantic scene. The feminine becomes consumptive because beauty itself is considered ill. Walter Pater in his essay on Leonardo Da Vinci concluded in that: "What may be called the fascination of corruption penetrates in every touch its exquisitely finished beauty" (Pater 1888, 129). According to Mario Praz, in *La carne, la muerte y el diablo en la literatura romántica,*

> el descubrimiento del horror, como fuente del deleite y de belleza, terminó por actuar sobre el mismo concepto de belleza: lo horrendo, en lugar de una categoría de lo bello, acabó por transformarse en uno de los elementos propios de la belleza. (1988, 69)

> The discovery of horror, as a source of delight and beauty, ended up acting on the very concept of beauty: the horrendous, instead of a category of the beautiful, ended up becoming one of the elements proper to beauty.

Yet Sontag emphasizes that TB grounds the link between death and aristocracy, since "remained the preferred way of giving death a meaning—an edifying, refined disease" (Sontag 1978, 16). In 1901, Antonio Espina y Capo notes that the intellectual consequences of consumption are:

> Hombres y mujeres, los tuberculosos, de lo más intelectuales dentro de su clase, aparecen en sociedad con un estado de lucidez notabilísimo: la mirada brillante, la palabra fácil, la concepción pronta; esto caracteriza el primer periodo de esta enfermedad. (Espina y Capo 1901, 109)

Men and women, tuberculosis patients, among the most intellectual within their class, appear in society with a remarkable state of lucidity: brilliant eyes, easy words, prompt conception; This characterizes the first period of this disease.

In Bécquer's words, there are a number of allusions to ruins that frequently invoke mystery, as in "La fe salva" (1969, 370). Characters are projected into ruins and assume their traits, as if they were a natural continuity of them. But the crumbling past is also reinstated as an image of the decomposing present. The consumptive is themselves a ruin from which a vestige of life ensues, much like a bastion or a fort abandoned to the mercy of the destructive power of nature. They operate as metaphors of decrepitude and are drawn as images of the appearance of the ill.

Consumption is part of a series of symptoms, such as anemia or chlorosis, qualified as "virgins' illness" by Helen King (2004). Alba del Pozo García concludes that "la tisis o tuberculosis viene además a constituirse en el síntoma futuro de una sexualidad mal regulada, aterradora y real consecuencia del eufemismo que refiere la clorosis" (García 2013, 117; Consumption or tuberculosis also becomes the future symptom of poorly regulated sexuality, terrifying and a real consequence of the euphemism that refers to chlorosis).

However, the diagnosis of TB obeys motifs that are sometimes opposed to one another: in some cases, the cause is attributed to all sorts of excess, while in others it is ascribed to absence, with an emphasis on the patient's virginity. Sontag points out that consumption works as a "way of describing sexual felling while lifting the responsibility of libertinism" while at the same time being "both a way of describing sensuality and promoting the claims of passion and a way of describing repression and advertising and promoting the claims of passion and a way of describing repression and advertising the claims of sublimation" (Sontag 1978, 24–25).

Within literature and art, TB operates as a plethora of meanings that allude both to the physical and to the moral realms. Symptoms are commonplace: paleness, eye bags, and cough convey a sensual, frail, delicate temper. One must only think of Clarín's story "El dúo de la tos," included in *Cuentos morales* (1896). These features were not exclusive to the ill but are instead a generalized expression of a delicate and sensitive spirit adjusted to aesthetic expectations. Bécquer starts "La fe salva" by emphasizing that

Encontrándome en el balneario de Fitero, en busca de un poco de salud para mi cuerpo dolorido y cansado, conocí a una mujer extraña de una dulce y marchita belleza. Representaba tener unos veinticinco años, aunque el sufrimiento, sin duda, había puesto en su rostro un sello de prematura vejez. (1969, 370)

Finding myself in the Fitero spa, in search of some health for my sore and tired body, I met a strange woman of a sweet and withered beauty. He represented to be about twenty-five years old, although suffering, without a doubt, had put on his face a stamp of premature old age.

TB was regarded as an illness of the spirit or the soul, since it was situated in the lungs, the noble and spiritual part of the body—another one of the links tying it to melancholy. With regards to TB, in *The Life and Adventures of Nicholas Nickleby*, Charles Dickens emphasizes that: "There is a dreaded disease which so prepares its victim, as it were, for death; which so refines it of its grosser aspect" (Dickens 1839, 565). The notion of a "dreaded disease" with a "refining" quality sheds light on contradictory desire, be it by excess or lack. Consumption is submitted to a mystifying process which yields the image of the sickly woman before yielding her truth. Fever caused by TB was considered a symptom of "internal scalding," expression of a "sickening love," and a "passion that consumes." For Romanticism, consumption is a "variant of the disease of love" (Sontag 1978, 20). The description of this illness often lacks a precise diagnosis, but one may conjecture from its symptoms that it is caused by consumption. The protagonist of "La fe salva" suffers from "inexplicable enfermedad que se prolongó, días y días, sin que nadie supiese lo que me pasaba," but, at the same time, her sister Blanca is said to be drawn to Alberto "como mariposas que abrasan, inconscientes, sus alas en la llama" (Bequer 1969, 374):

> inexplicable disease that lasted, days and days, without anyone knowing what was happening to me, but, at the same time, her sister Blanca are said to be drawn to Alberto like butterflies that burn, unconscious, their wings on the calls. (Bequer 1969, 374)

It is important to note that the illness, in its literary portrayal, is often conveyed in enigmatic terms, without a known attributable cause to a series of symptoms. Nevertheless, when the symptoms are fragility, languor, and weakness physically translated in eye bags and paleness, TB is implied. Sontag adds,

> TB was understood, like insanity, to be a kind of one-sideness: a failure of Will or an overintensity. However much the disease was dreads, TB always had pathos. Like the mental patient today, the tubercular was considered to be someone quintessentially vulnerable, and full of self-destructive whims. (Sontag 1978, 63–64)

The image of the ill woman, and of the non-ill woman, recovers striking actuality and favors its transformation into a literary topic. At times it seems as if the poets fall in love with the same image, independently of its concrete feminine embodiment. This impulse may be explained as stemming from the shared image of universal valency of a feminine type against the grain of reality. Beauty is only beauty if it fades. The final stanza of Bécquer's XI rhyme suggests the same context:

> Yo soy un sueño, un imposible, aquía\Vano fantasma de niebla
> y luz,
> Soy incorpórea, soy intangible, (412)

> An empty phantom of mist and light;
> I am ethereal, I am intangible;

TB is a necessary condition of the process. It is not merely what explains the foreseeable disappearing, but what cyphers the sense of beauty itself. Consumption seduces because there are occasions in which death coexists with the semblance of life. Consumptive beauty is literally untouchable, inaccessible, but it is beauty precisely because it is inaccessible, impalpable, and untouchable. Rhyme XX illustrates love as conditioned by illness, even if not necessarily referring to it.

> Sabe, si alguna vez tus labios rojos
> Quema invisible atmósfera abrasada,

> If your red lips are ever heated
> by an invisible burst of air, ("Gustavo Adolfo Bécquer—Rimas")

This is the case, in part, because of the consumptive's self-involvement since, in reality, the consumptive already transits the world as a living-dead. For Susan Sontag, "The Romantics moralized death in a new way: with the TB death, which dissolved the gross body, etherealized the personality, expanded consciousness" (1978, 19). Reality fosters fictionalization because it cannot be captured through any other means. Figuration is not a matter of choosing between a plethora of possibilities, but of taking on the only alternative. Capturing reality is only possible when accepting the impossibility of it. The making of the unmakeable. This paradox guards the romantic tragedy in which the artist appears as split—without the possibility of reconciliation—from not feminine beauty but from the artist themselves. This caesura opens the door to melancholy: "the melancholic primarily suffers from the contradiction between time and infinite, while at the same time giving a positive value to his own sorrow 'sub specie aeternitatis,' since he feels that through his very melancholy he has a share in eternity" (Klibansky, Panofsky, and Fritz 1979, 235). Melancholy exacerbates its own symptoms before consumption, with which it shares the intimate contradiction between a sense of finitude and infinitude. The consumptive seems to notice, in the melancholic, a victim of the same suffering but in the moral order. The melancholic's conflict between the ephemeral and the eternal is similar, with some caveats, to the certainty of the consumptive's foreseeable death. Rhyme LXVI invoques such a relationship:

> ¿Adónde voy?
> El más sombrío y triste
>
> Where am I going?
> the saddest wasteland ("Gustavo Adolfo Bécquer—Rimas")

Melancholy comes forth through sadness, indicative of a sensible and refined temper. In the sixteenth century, there was already a likeness drawn between both afflictions, according to Klibansky, Panofsky, and Saxl: "the fusion of the characters 'Melancholy' and 'Tristesse' during the fifteenth century brought about not only a modification of the notion of Melancholy, in the sense of giving it a subjective vagueness, but also, *vice versa*, of the notion of grif, giving it the connotations of brooding thoughtfulness and quasi-pathological refinements" (Klibansky, Panofsky, and Saxl 1979, 231). Much like TB, melancholy intensifies self-awareness. Throughout the nineteenth century, it immediately invoked sickly beauty. In a passage from his *Journaux intimes*, Charles Baudelaire notes: "Je ne prétends pas que la Joie ne puisse pas s'associer avec la Beauté, mais je dis que la Joie est un des ornements les plus vulgaires, tandis que la Mélancolie en est pour ainsi dire l'illustre compagne, à ce point que je ne conçois guère (mon cerveau serait-il un miroir ensorcelé ?) un type de Beauté où il n'y ait du Malheur" (1880, 20). The link with sadness becomes evident in rhyme LXVIII:

> No sé lo que he soñado
> en la noche pasada; (445)
>
> I do not know what
> I dreamed last night; ("Gustavo Adolfo Bécquer—Rimas")

In the first letter written related to *Desde mi celda*, Becquer refers to a melancholic state as inseparable from TB as cause of the spleen that possesses him:

Yo he oído decir a muchos, y aun la experiencia me ha enseñado un poco, que hay horas peligrosas, horas lentas y cargadas de extraños pensamientos y de una voluptuosa pesadez, contra las que es imposible defenderse; es esas horas, como cuando nos turban la cabeza los vapores del vino, los sonidos se debilitan y parece que se oyen muy distantes, los objetos se ven como velados por una gasa azul, y el deseo presta audacia al espíritu, que recobra para sí todas las fuerzas que pierde la materia. (1969, 507)

I have heard many say, and experience has even taught me a little, that there are dangerous hours, slow hours charged with strange thoughts and a voluptuous heaviness, against which it is impossible to defend oneself; It is those hours, as when the vapors of wine trouble our heads, the sounds weaken and seem to be heard very distant, the objects are seen as veiled by a blue gauze, and desire lends audacity to the spirit, which recovers for itself all the forces that matter loses.

He associates these dreamy moments with dawn, by drawing on characteristics that are not far from those of the meridian demon lurking in the afternoon hours, a formula which refers to the "acedia, tristitia, taedium vitae, desídia" (Agamben 1995, 23). These states of mind are favorable to melancholia and in Bécquer's lines correlate to some effects of the meridian demon referred to by Giorgio Agamben:

torpor, el obtuso y somnoliento estupor que paraliza cualquier gesto que pudiera curarnos; y finalmente *evagatio mentis*, la fuga del ánimo ante sí mismo y el inquieto discurrir de fantasía en fantasía que se manifiesta en la *verbositas*, la monserga vanamente proliferante sobre sí mismo, en la curiositas, la insaciable sed de ver por ver que se dispersa en posibilidades siempre nuevas, en la *instabilitas loci vel propositi* y en la *importunitas mentis*, la petulante incapacidad de fijar en un orden y un ritmo el propio pensamiento. (1995, 27–28)

torpor, the obtuse and sleepy stupor that paralyzes any gesture that could heal us; and finally evagatio mentis, the flight of the mind before itself and the restless flow from fantasy to fantasy that manifests itself in the verbositas, the vainly proliferating nonsense about itself, in the curiositas, the insatiable thirst to see to see that disperses in ever new possibilities, in the instabilitas loci vel propositi and in the importunitas mentis, the petulant inability to fix thought itself in order and rhythm.

Among the possible remedies to cure TB, it was believed that the ill should be isolated from the community. Separation exacerbates individuality. The individual is confronted with themselves, separated, alienated, emancipated as they are from the others. This is a sort of banishing or forced exile caused by the illness and brought about by medical prescription rather than by the patient's will.

In a letter signed in Soria in March 1861, Bécquer confides to his friend Ramón Rodríguez Correa:

Mañana emprendemos el camino de Veruela. ¡Ojalá el viejo monasterio me dé calma y la resignación que necesito, pues mi alma es un pobre guiñapo insensible, dormido, que me pesa como un fardo inútil que la fatalidad tiró sobre mis hombros, y con el cual me obliga a caminar como un nuevo judío errante! En el amplio hogar de la cocina me entretuve anoche en quemar todas las cartas, únicos recuerdos -reliquias, mejor dicho- que me quedaban de mi vida de ayer, de las horas que nunca volverán. Al enroscarse a los rotos pliegues la llama, parecía su mano, una mano amarilla, de muerte, que se burlaba de mí. Haciendo signos incomprensibles; aquella mano que hoy estará prisionera entre otras. No quiero pensar nada, sentir nada. (Padilla 2004)

Tomorrow we start the road to Veruela. Hopefully the old monastery will give me calm and the resignation I need, for my soul is a poor, insensitive, sleeping rag that weighs me down like a useless burden that fate has thrown on my shoulders, and with which it forces me to walk like a new wandering jew! In the large hearth in the kitchen last night I amused myself by burning all the letters, the only memories -relics, rather- that I had left from my life from yesterday, from the hours that will never come back. As the flame coiled around the torn folds, it seemed like her hand, a yellow hand, of death, that mocked me. Making incomprehensible signs; that hand that today will be a prisoner among others. I don't want to think anything, feel anything.

This description, from 1864, is a conventional depiction of melancholic temper, but it introduces the variable of illness, which gives sincerity to it. The place outstands due to its geographic height and harsh weather, prescribed by doctors in order to combat the alleged "humidity of the lungs" caused by TB. Both the landscape and melancholic temper align with the suffering of TB suggesting a sentiment of infinite. Honoré de Balzac stops at the ruins in *Médecin de campagne* (1800):

Pourquoi les hommes ne regardent-ils point sans une émotion profonde toutes les ruines, même les plus humbles? Sans doute, elles sont pour eux une image du malheur dont le poids est senti par eux si diversement. Les cimetières font penser à la mort, un village abandonné fait songer aux peines de la vie; la mort est un malheur prévu, les peines de la vie sont infinies. L'infini n'est-il pas le secret des grandes mélancolies? (48)

Why do men not look without deep emotion at all ruins, even the most humble? No doubt they are for them an image of misfortune, the weight of which is felt by them so differently. The cemeteries make one think of death, an abandoned village makes one think of the pains of life; death is an expected misfortune, the pains of life are endless. Isn't the infinite the secret of great melancholy?

Ruins constitute the remains of an abolished time, a substitute of eternity. Social banishing operates as justification for a wandering in search of natural surroundings appropriate for healing. The consumpted is thus transformed into nomad. They do not only wander from place to place, but hikes and expeditions are incorporated to their routine. For the writer, these journeys arouse curiosity. Bécquer indicates in the third missive:

> Hace dos o tres días, andando a la casualidad por entre estos montes, y habiéndome alejado más de lo que acostumbro en mis paseos matinales, acerté a descubrir, casi oculto entre las quiebras del terreno y fuera de todo camino, un pueblecillo cuya situación, por extremo pintoresca, me agradó tanto, que no pude por menos de aproximarme a él para examinar a mis anchas. (1969, 527)

> Two or three days ago, walking by chance among these mountains, and having strayed further than I am used to in my morning walks, I happened to discover, almost hidden among the breaks in the terrain and out of the way, a small town whose situation is extremely picturesque, I liked it so much that I could not help but approach it to examine it to my heart's content.

Thus, TB was received as a death certificate. The pain from which the melancholic suffered strived for an infinite that, for the tisic, has a prescribed date. There is nothing more natural than being attracted to ruins as expression of their own present. Melancholy, vagrancy, ruins, and death are elements inseparable from the Romantic vision associated with TB. In his letter III, Becquér complements:

> Cuando, no sin tener que forcejear antes un poco, logré abrir la carcomida y casi deshecha puerta del pequeño cementerio que por casualidad había encontrado en mi camino, y aquel se ofreció a mi vista, no pude menos de confiarme a mis ideas. Es imposible ni aun concebir un sitio más agreste, más solitario y más triste, con una agradable tristeza, que aquel. Nada habla allí de la muerte con ese lenguaje enfático y pomposo de los epitafios, nada la recuerda de modo que horrorice con el repugnante espectáculo de sus atavíos y despojos. . . . Al pie de las tapias, y por entre sus rendijas, crecen la hiedra y esas campanillas de color rosa pálido que suben sosteniéndose en las asperezas del muro hasta trepar a los bardales de heno, por donde se cruzan y se mecen como una flotante guirnalda de verdura. (1969, 529–30)

> When, not without having to struggle a little before, I managed to open the rotten and almost broken door of the small cemetery that I had found by chance on my way, and that one offered itself to my sight, I could not help trusting myself to my ideas. It is impossible to even conceive of a more wild, lonelier and sadder place, with a pleasant sadness, than that. Nothing there speaks of death with that emphatic and pompous language of epitaphs, nothing remembers it in such a

way that it horrifies with the disgusting spectacle of its finery and spoils. . . . At the foot of the walls, and through their cracks, ivy grows. and those pale-pink bluebells that climb, holding on to the roughness of the wall, until they climb the hay bales, where they intersect and sway like a floating garland of greens.

For the Romantic self, nothing is left untouched. But if something represents the ideal of beauty, it is the ill feminine that concentrates all of these senses. Love doubly avoids the woman in love since the consumpted woman is inaccessible due to her illness but, mainly, because her faith is imminent death. Both circumstances impulse idealism as an option of realization. Love nests exclusively in the ideal. Mystification is resolved into ideal contrary to reality. Sickness excludes from society whoever suffers from it, but at the same time it does so with the lover of the beloved. The image of woman becomes sublimated. This process explains the fact that most women poetized by Romantic authors share similar features, commonly associated to physical and moral symptoms of TB: vulnerability and fragility, spirituality and evanescence, tragedy and death. In reality, reciprocity between the poet's sensibility—occasionally also suffering from TB—and the consumpted woman as object of love was usually fostered. The relationship was established from the acknowledgment of a temper that participated of meanings associated with TB. Consumption operates as an adjusted metaphor of Romanticism. At first glance, it is surprising that beauty belongs in a principle of physical corruption signified by the languor of consumption. It is about a first stage that results in the *femme fatal* of the end of the century, in which moral transgression no longer requires physical annihilation but has the same cause. Diderot had written in his letter to Sophie Vollan on July 18, 1762:

> Presque toujours ce qui nuit à la beauté morale redouble la beauté poétique. On ne fait guère que des tableaux tranquilles et froids avec la vertu; c'est la passion et le vice qui animent les compositions du peintre, du poète et du musicien.

> Almost always what harms moral beauty redoubles poetic beauty. We only paint calm and cold pictures with virtue; it is passion and vice that animate the compositions of the painter, the poet and the musician.

CONCLUSION

Gustavo Adolfo Bécquer's oeuvre is inseparable from TB as expression of Romantic imaginary. It does not project only toward feminine beauty but toward himself. The symptoms of this illness surround its structure without necessarily referring to it explicitly, though it seems that in some way or another it constantly alludes to consumption. Actually, there is an overlap.

It is not only about the author's suffering but about the appropriation of a Romantic metaphor as slogan. TB generated feminine beauty features in Romanticism but at the same time its associated senses are meaningful. Ruins and mystery favor an idealism at service of the inaccessible. When in the physical the ruling are the symptoms of TB, in morality melancholy irrupts as a persistent state, inseparable from illness. Both conditions prelude the end of the century's tedium. Bécquer's work does not only predictably adjust to its time, but encloses some of the elements that will later equip Decadentism. It is still not morbid, but morbidity is already present in his writing. He is still not an erotic writer and yet eroticism slides into his writing. He's still not decadent, but decaying elements are undeniably present. Bécquer gives meaning to Hispanic Romanticism, but also inaugurates a budding modernity. It seems that the sense of his work is inseparable from the figuration and sublimation of TB.

NOTES

1. All quotes from Bécquer's works come from the 1969 edition. All of the English translations were translated by Mercedes Zavala.

REFERENCES

Agamben, Giorgio. *Estancias. La palabra y el fantasma en la cultura occidental.* Translated by Tomás Segovia. Valencia: Pre-Textos, 1995.
Argullol, Rafael. *La atracción del abismo. Un itinerario por el paisaje romántico.* Barcelona: Plaza y Janés, 1987.
Balzac, Honoré de. *Médecin de campagne.* Paris: Bibliothèque Larousse, 1800.
Baudelaire, Charles. *Journaux intimes. Fusées. Mon cœur mis à nu.* Paris: Les Éditions G. Crès et Cie, 1880.
Bécquer, Gustavo Adolfo. *Obras completas.* Madrid: Aguilar, 1969.
Colli, Giorgio. *Apolíneo y dinosíaco.* Translated by Miguel Morey and edited by Enrico Colli. México: SextoPiso, 2020.
Covarrubias, Miguel de. *Tesoro de la lengua castellana o española.* Barcelona: Altafulla, 1998.
D'Aurevilly, Barbey. *Léa.* Paris: La Connaissance, 1921.
Dalí, Salvador. "Le surréalisme spectral de l'éternel féminin préraphaélite." *Minotaure* 8 (1936): 45–49.
Dickens, Charles. *The Life and Adventures of Nicholas Nickleby.* London: Champman and Hall, 1839.
Diderot, Denis. *L'Encyclopédie, ou Dictionnaire raisonné des sciences, des arts et des matiers.* Paris, 1751.

Espina y Capo, Antonio. *Estudio de climoterapia e higiene del enfermo en esta estación:Panticosa, pirineos españoles*. Madrid: Asilo de Huérfanos del Sagrado Corazón de Jesús, 1901.

Flaubert, Gustave. *Correspondance. Anné 1853*. 1853. https://flaubert.univrouen.fr/correspondance/conard/outils/1853.htm

Grellet, Isabelle, and Caroline Kruse. *Histoires de la tuberculose. Les fièvres de l'âme 18001940*. Paris: Ramsayd, 1983.

Jacobsen, J. P. *Mogens and Other Stories*. Create Space Independent Publishing Plataform, 2017.

King, Helen. *The Disease of Virgins: Green Sickness, Chorosis and the Problems of Puberty*. London: Routledge, 2004.

Klibansky, Raymond, Erwin Panofsky, and Fritz Saxel. *Saturn and Melancholy*. The Netherlands, 1979.

Litvak, Lily. *Erotismo fin de siglo*. Barcelona: Bosch, 1979.

Padilla, José Monteiro. "Bécquer em Veruela." Centro Virtual Cervantes. 2004. https://cvc.cervantes.es/el_rinconete/anteriores/julio_04/07072004_02.htm

Pater, Walter. *The Renaissence. Studies in Art and Poetry*. London: MacMillan, 1888.

Pozo García, Alba del. *Género y enfermedad en la literatura española del fin de siglo XIXXX*. Barcelona: Tesis de doctorado, 2013.

Praz, Mario. *El pacto con la serpiente. Paralipómenos de "La carne, la muerte y el diabloen la literatura romántica."* Translated by Ida Vitale. México: Fondo de Cultura Económica, 1988.

Praz, Mario. *La carne, la muerte y el diablo en la literatura romántica*. Translated by Rubén Mettini. Barcelona: El Acantilado, 1999.

Pulido, Ángel. *Bosquejos médico-sociales para la mujer*. Madrid: Víctor Sainz, 1876.

Rossetti, Dante Gabriel. *The Works of Dante Gabriel Rossetti*. London: Ellis, 1911.

Sontag, Susan. *Illness as a Metaphor*. New York: Farrar, Straus and Giroux, 1978.

Chapter Two

The Turn of the Century and the Spanish Imaginary Facing the Disease

The Case of Ganivet

Ricardo de la Fuente Ballesteros and Juan R. Coca

The fields of medicine and, more specifically, psychiatry were aware, during the nineteenth century, that the human mind was affected by volition and will. These factors could come to condition human behavior and fall into the psychological construct called apathy (Berrios and Gili 1995). This concept was related, to a greater or lesser degree, to the existence of social, economic, and collective health problems. In fact, Kupperman (1979) indicates that the high mortality rates in the United States of America during the seventeenth century also generated psychological effects such as apathy. Well, during the nineteenth century, apathy had so much social impact that Ángel Ganivet himself developed, for the first time, the concept of abulia to designate a disease of these characteristics; illness which, on the other hand, was diffuse and imprecise. Hence, Berrios and Gili (1995) consider that it is maintained today and defend its designation as diseases of the will, similar to what Ribot had already exposed in his *Les maladies de la volonté* in 1984 (Jurkevich 1992).

Melancholy, as László Földényi (2016) repeatedly points out, has been present in the history of human thought. However, not in all epochs did this condition have the same impact. Ehrenreich (2008) wrote that in the Baroque period there was an epidemic of melancholy. However, the concept of melancholy has been full of conjectures and indefinition throughout human history. In fact, the vague and diffuse idea of melancholy is related to the theory of humors, born in ancient Greece, so much so that melancholy was related to black bile. This conception was maintained until the eighteenth century, when it was transformed into a neurophysiological explanation. In this sense, Anne-Charles Lorry differentiated in 1765 between *mélancolie humorale* and *mélancolie nerveuse*, which shows a certain transformation in the meaning of the term. Lorry also indicated that nervous melancholy is related to the limitations of reality and human desires. Therefore, modern melancholy (and its derivatives such as abulia) was, in part, related to volition at first. Gradually, however, the idea that the will, understood as a mental construct, was the cause of this type of affliction became less and less important at the end of the nineteenth century. However, we will focus on this period and its transition to the twentieth century to understand, thanks to Ganivet, some aspects of the conceptual evolution of melancholy or abulia.

The transit between the nineteenth and the twentieth centuries, commonly known as the "la fin du siècle," was an enormously highlighted moment in the history of the European continent. This historical moment coincides with the great migratory exodus from Europe to the United States. This mass immigration, mostly from the south of Europe, took place due to the agrarian crisis together with social and religious conflicts, as well as political revolutions. These crises together were represented by the literature in what is conventionally called hyper-romanticism (Herman 1998, 52). However, the main triggers of this social phenomenon were the demographic and economic conditions of the regions where most of the migrants lived (Comín 2012, 456). In this changing situation characterized by different conflicts, it is not surprising that the theories on human degeneration were implemented mainly based on social Darwinism.

Social Darwinism, after all, was the most prominent term that better marked the sense of crisis that existed at that time. Crisis immersed in a communal, organicist, and collectivist conception as each one prefers to understand it. At that time, the idea of society as the organism of organisms was notorious (González Serrano 1884, 89). Nevertheless, the studies of Max Nordau[1] on physiology and mental diseases were also of an outstanding relevance. Max Nordau is undoubtedly one of the great milestones of this field. This author achieves, with his book *Degeneration*[2] (1892) a notable impact on the society of his time, as well as on the writers and artists of that moment. Pio Baroja himself indicated that it was an insane work and that he had imagined himself in a madhouse (Baroja 1899, 33). Influenced by positivism, criminal sociology, and social Darwinism, Nordau based his analysis on an organicist vision that led him to fight for a society that was not decadent and, therefore could escape from "moral madness, imbecility and insanity" (Nordau 1902, 9).

In a summarized way, it was believed that this "sick" and "decadent" society could be avoided (Bergua 2019, 21–23). One of the characteristics of modernity was at first the separation between the natural and the social.

To this was added the well-known secularism and the desire for intervention. These characteristics began to take shape in the earlier Baroque era (Soldevilla 2013, 54). In the Renaissance, the tearing of the self began to unravel little by little. It led to a certain configuration of therapeutics in society, as the Bildungsroman (the novel of training or learning) demonstrates well. In any case, this is not the time to delve into these issues; just keep in mind that the "pathological" characteristics of modernity were already an intrinsic part of the culture (as is often the case).

These basic elements are the wicks of the industrial explosion that brought progress, work, but also conflict and health problems. Precisely for this last reason, an approach within the world of biomedicine began to stand out: the hygienic vision of society. In general, these ideas were deeply concerned about the phenomenon of social health and the improvement of people's lives. But, as always happens, within this concept there was also a strong imprint of the mechanisms of moralization.

The hygienist tendencies were united, in one way or another, with the approaches of the business bourgeoisie at that time. The concept of hygiene and the concept of morality ended up being two fundamental pillars of the so-called Social Medicine (Campos 1995). We find here one of the expressions of the will that characterizes modernity expressed by a principle that nothing is more than an incorporation of reality in the imaginary (Bergua 2019, 37). By facing social decadence, medical science stands as the ability to provide solutions and establish adequate morality. Therefore, we are before an episteme or an impulse based on the medicalization of society, in which the concept of decadence is understood as a stigmatizing phenomenon and in a "botched civilization" (Pine 1988, 24). This deliquesce today has been mentioned, in one way or another, by different numbers of sociologists such as Luis Enrique Alonso, George Balandier, Zygmunt Bauman, José Ángel Bergua, Josetxo Beriaín, and Juan Antonio Roche, to mention just a few. All of them have shown the social ambivalence of these different ideas such as control/freedom, fraternity violence, and information/misinformation. An interesting example of this can be found in Antoine Compagnon's (2005) *Les antimodernes de Joseph de Maistre à Roland Barthes*, which defines the dandy as an anti-modern, although the dandy is close to an aristocratic and heraldic conception (Pine 1998) that reveals itself against the deliquescent evolution of history. Now, the dandy, after all, is part of that modern ambivalence and is, therefore, a modern phenomenon.

Let us return to the scope of the degeneration relating now to Ángel Ganivet. Like most of the Ibero-American writers at that moment, he incorporated the identification of social degeneration with illness, emphasizing its negative connotations. Hence, he stands against the patriotic cause of such an element. He proclaims that degeneration is a phenomenon that comes from

France and does not have anything to do with the Spanish spirit. The same ambiguity is found in the Hispano-American writers in Europe. Degeneration and decadence, they emphasized, was something that did not match their youth; only by imitation they can be infected. As Darío says in "Después del Carnaval" (After Carnival):

> Europa tiene necesidad de excitantes para el goce, como los viejos fatigados. Y América imita y sigue todo lo Europeo; nosotros, pueblos jóvenes, imitamos los gestos de allá, nos inoculamos la enfermedad de allá. (Ganivet 1943, IV, 771)[3]

> Europe has a need for excitement like old fatigued. And America imitates them and follows all Europeans; we, young people, imitate their gestures. We inoculate ourselves with their diseases. (Ganivet 1943, IV, 771)

Again, we find ourselves with some ambivalence in authors such as Ruben Darío or Gómez Carrillo. Both are deeply interested in degenerated characters and diseases, which are related, in one way or another, with creativity and mental brilliance. From a social perspective, degeneration is conceived as negative and, therefore, avoidable (de la Fuente Ballesteros 2001; 2007; Cardwell 1998). These ideas form part of an episteme that has been built since antiquity in which the artist deviates from the normality and which was generated in the nineteenth century from Moreau de Tours in his works, *De la influence du Physique sur la moral* (1830), *Les facultés morales* (1836), and *La psychologie morbide* (1859). All of them portray the concept of "superior degenerates" applied to the relationship between genius and madness, which will be expanded by the works of Cesare Lombroso where the element of pathology is strengthened to scrutinize the artist. These ideas are related to his works *Genio e follia* (1864), *L'uomo di genio* (1888), and *Genio e degenerazione* (1897).

In short, the concern for illness and for the conception that society is gradually degenerating became a constant in a nourished group of authors. In turn, this increase in the theme of illness in discourse brings with it the difference between social class differences affected by this imagination in biomedical terms. A terminological change was even carried out which indicates, in addition to social concern, superiority of the physician. Examples are emphasized through terms which have moral connotative elements such the words drunk and drunkenness, which were gradually replaced by more biomedical ones such as alcoholism.

Another element of great importance for the future debates is related to the concept of normality (Foucault 2001). Previously, it used to be about health issues in general, but at the end of twentieth and the beginning of the twentieth-first century, has generated a remarkable amount of specialized bibliography. Regarding the words normal and abnormal, Rafael Huertas García-Alejo (1987) clearly explains that they were related to the theories of degeneration, which were used by psychiatry and medicine. This concept of normality, despite its positivist character in relation to statistical normality, is an abstract and arbitrary term that dominant groups used to turn into abnormal everything that is not located within the instituted imagination. In order words, the concepts of normality and abnormality were used to maintain the power in the hands of the bourgeoisie. The artists and writers were placed in a marginal position.

APATHY IN GANIVET'S WORK

Ganivet was not a writer who was outside the social and the historical contexts in which he lived. He also incorporated the positivist imaginary of the medicalization of the society of his time, which has been shown by other researchers (Pick 1999; Nye 1984). In his first work, *España filosófica contemporánea y otros trabajos*, he identified positivism as the evil in his homeland (Ganivet 1930). Skepticism toward science was generic in most of these artists. Thus, we read in Miguel Unamuno:

> El escepticismo hacia la ciencia es algo genérico en la mayoría de estos artistas. Así leemos en Unamuno: "¡El cientificismo . . . es la plaga de la inteligencia" (Unamuno 1968 . . . , 914), o "¡Progresar por progresar, llegar a la ciencia del bien y del mal para hacernos dioses! Todo esto no es más que avaricia, forma concreta de toda idolatría, hacer de los medios fines." (Unamuno 1929, 231–32)

> "Scientism . . . is the plague of intelligence" (Unamuno 1968, 914), or "Progress by progressing, reaching the science of good and good! Bad to make us gods! All this, is nothing more than greed, a concrete form of all idolatry, making means ends." (Unamuno 1929, 231–32)

The Basque writer, like many modernist writers, subscribed to his distrust of the worldview of continuous progress. In a growing context of the explosion of science,[4] he also shared the irrationality with the majority of his generation. In the same way, Díaz Rodríguez raises in his custody the emblem of Alonso Quijano, "el caballero divino cuya locura destella sobre el juicio reposado y trivial del vulgo" (the divine knight whose madness shines on the quiet and trivial judgment of the vulgar) (Díaz 1942, 61) and explodes against the substitution that was made at the time by the cult of science versus religion; what's more, what happened, from his point of view, is that one had been substituted for the other (Díaz 1942, 68–71).

All this is not new, since the germ of these attitudes of resistance are already found in Baudelaire, who in Universal Exhibition-1855-Fine Arts is dispatched on the idea of progress on which adjectives such as "grotesque" is opposed to the love for the beauty that no longer has a place in this society. He asks:

> ¿Cuál es la garantía del progreso para el futuro? Porque los discípulos de los filósofos del vapor y de las cerillas químicas no conciben el progreso sino bajo la forma de una serie indefinida. ¿Dónde está entonces, esa garantía?, para concluir: "Yo afirmo que sólo en vuestra credulidad y fatuidad.

> What is the guarantee of progress for the future? Because the disciples of the philosophers of steam and chemical matches do not conceive progress except in the form of an indefinite series. Where is that guarantee then? To conclude: "I affirm that only in your credulity and fatuity). (Baudelaire 2000, 1207–08).

In "Nuevos Apuntes" about Edgar Allan Poe, Baudelaire says:

> ¿No es tema de asombro que no estalle en todos los cerebros esta idea tan sencilla: que el Progreso (mientras haya progreso) perfecciona el dolor en la proporción en que refina el placer, y que, si la epidermis de los pueblos se va delicadizando [*sic*], evidentemente no están persiguiendo sino una *Italia fugientem*, una conquista perdida a cada minuto, un progreso siempre negador de sí mismo? (Baudelaire 2000, 909)

> Is it not a matter of astonishment that this simple idea does not explode in all brains: that Progress (while there is progress) perfects pain in proportion as it refines pleasure, and that, if the skin of the peoples is becoming more delicate [sic], obviously they are not pursuing but a fugitive Italy, a lost conquest every minute, a progress always denying itself? (Baudelaire 2000, 909)

This position of the French poet denotes that in his denial of the Good he is also denying the priority of the future. What he puts on the table is the paralysis of modern man in the face of a modernity conceived as progress (Bataille 1957, 45–49).

This imaginary arises as a reaction to an increased number of social problems produced by industrialization and the conflicts of the time. For this reason, for many authors, the nation (a concept that also takes on unusual importance from this moment on) was undergoing a process of degradation. In the Ganivetian work entitled *Idearium Español* (1897), we can verify this same conviction of which we have just spoken. The Spanish nation is in a situation of dramatic transit due to the "abatimiento patológico" (pathological dejection) (de la Fuente Ballesteros 1998) whose main cause *es el no-querer* (is not wanting to). This concept could be translated by the anomie, and about it Emile Durkheim spoke in 1933 in his *De la division du travail social* (1991) with a great impact on later sociology. Let's see how the words that Ganivet expresses in this sense:

> Si yo fuese consultado como médico espiritual para formular el diagnóstico del padecimiento que los españoles sufrimos . . . diría que la enfermedad que se designa con el nombre de "no-querer" o, en términos más científicos, por la palabra griega *aboulia*. (Ganivet 1943, I, 226)

> If I were consulted as a spiritual doctor to formulate the diagnosis of the condition that we Spaniards suffer . . . I would say that the disease that is designated by the name of "not-wanting" or, in more scientific terms, by the Greek word aboulia. (Ganivet 1943, I, 226)

This concept of aboulia (abulia) (Arjona 1928; Jurkevich 1992; Láscaris 1952; Senabre 1974; Ramsden 1974; Shaw 1997; Ardila 2007) is characterized, according to our author, as "the extinction or serious weakening of the will," which has its organic cause in mental disorders. Ganivet, as criticized by different authors such as Azaña (1921, 94) or Ortega y Gasset (1946), did not delve too deeply into the importance of apathy at the social level and, furthermore, it seems that the author's intention was more than anything to characterize what he understood to be the Spanish society of the time. After all, he affirmed that society is the result of the sum of individual wills. Hence, for him, psychology could provide knowledge of existing social pathology. In this sense, it is extremely shocking that, from an individualistic perspective, a national evil was established as if we were talking about an infection. According to Ganivet, Spanish society as a whole did not use intelligence to establish associations thanks to it. This lack in the use of this faculty in a chronic way is what causes such a condition (Ganivet 1897).

These ideas were their own at the time. In fact, we can find something similar to apathy in what Unamuno raised when he spoke of unwillingness.[5] Both authors focus their interest on the Spanish territory; it seems that their proposal could not be extended to the rest of society, something that Durkheim did. Perhaps this limited the possible expansion of the idea, although this is still a question without a possible answer.

The person who is affected by apathy has a lack of intellectual will, spiritual lethargy, inability to concentrate and learn, etc. But what are the reasons for this apathy? Ganivet mentions purely psychic causes. In the first place, it refers to the studies on insanity and the investigations of the alienists. In fact, Ángel Ganivet indicates in his *Idearium español* (Spanish Idearium, 1897) that his analysis of the concept of apathy is based on individual psychological models. According to him, apathy produces a lack of spirit to carry out actions, inaction, which we could say goes against the spirit of the human being. However, Ganivet leaves aside the socio-occupational situation of apathetic person, contrary to the doctors of the time who actively intervened to soften the conflict and improve the sanitation of the workers' environment (Campos 1997). Once these elements have been explained, Ganivet focuses his interest on showing the differences between nations with the capacity to, he says, "act consciously, to know their own destinies well" and nations in which "disagreement predominates; partial interests, which are like isolated representations in individuals" (1897, 124). We find, then, a gap in the process of understanding the sociological phenomenon of apathy and an absence in the answer that we raised before.

Ganivet, son of his time, manifests his romantic and platonic[6] stamp when trying to solve the conflict in relation to apathy. According to him, there are "intelligent and disinterested" people (Ganivet 1897, 133) who could lead the "combat" in order to "restore spiritual life." These Ganivetian considerations no doubt remind the government of the Platonic philosophers in that they would be able to come out of the cave and tell the prisoners who are still inside the reality that is outside. An intellectual aristocracy that was also promoted in the artistic movement of Romanticism (Cordova). However, Ganivet fails to see that people's social conditions affect their psychic conditioning factors, something that Durkheim is able to detect. In addition, Ganivet does not seem to be aware that the living conditions of the people also affect the capacities of the subjects. In fact, Ganivet makes no mention of anything like it. His individualism did not make him aware of such a possibility, although his text, in relation to apathy, has a markedly socio-political character, so much so that he goes so far as to affirm that societies also have personality, which is why this social disease of apathy is embedded in that collective Spanish personality.

On the other hand, Ganivet speaks of himself as suffering from apathy—inserted also in environmental pathologization (Aronna 1993; Ramsden 1967, 125):

> Hay una forma vulgar de la abulia que todos conocemos y a veces padecemos. ¿A quién no le habrá invadido en alguna ocasión esa perplejidad de espíritu, nacida del quebranto de fuerzas o del aplanamiento consiguiente a una inacción prolongada, en que la voluntad, falta de una idea dominante que la mueva, vacilante entre motivos opuestos que se contrabalancean, o dominada por una idea abstracta, irrealizable, permanece irresoluta, sin saber qué hacer y sin determinarse a hacer nada? (Ganivet 1943, I, 226–27)

> There is a vulgar form of apathy that we all know and sometimes suffer from. Who has not ever been invaded by that perplexity of spirit, born of the

breakdown of forces or the flattening resulting from prolonged inaction, in which the will, lacking a dominant idea to move it, vacillating between opposing motives that are counterbalanced, or dominated by an abstract, unrealizable idea, remains unsolved, without knowing what to do and without determining to do anything? (Ganivet 1943, I, 226–27)

In the private correspondence written by Ganivet himself, it is clear that he too felt that this disease affected him. In fact, in a letter written in 1893 he states the following: "Every day, it becomes more difficult for me to concentrate my ideas and fix my thoughts on a specific object" (Ganivet 1943, II, 811). In a second letter written in 1894, he again makes a certain reference to the lack of energy. This time he even goes so far as to associate it with a certain sexual frustration. We cannot say that this fact is surprising. George H. Mead in his work *Spirit, Person and Society* (1982) clearly shows us the interrelationship between the societal and the personal. The consciousness of a society, he tells us, is organized around the subject. This is so since the experience that each of us has as a person is an experience received as a function of action with others. For this reason, Ganivet's study also allows us to understand some of the aspects of society and the historical moment of that moment. One of them is precisely that ambivalence or paradox of some of the authors who followed the theory of degeneration and who spoke of social disease. At the end of the day, the moral rigor and biological determinism that permeated the theoretical proposal of degeneration also produced a certain clash with the life-world of its promoters. We wonder if the contradictions posed by this vision also affected Ganivet.

GANIVET IN THE INS AND OUTS OF THE WILL

We have indicated before that the Spanish writer presented his proposal of apathy as a characterizing element of the Spain of his time. Now, reading his work leads one to conclude that he relied on his own life experience to develop his proposal. We have already indicated that, on some occasions, Ganivet said of himself that he was affected by apathy. After all, Ganivet focused his interest on reason and will in a similar way to Schopenhauer (de la Fuente Ballesteros 1996; Santibáñez Tió 1994, 81). Although Ganivet states in the *Idearium* (1897) that his study on apathy was based on individual psychological models (derived from clinical cases), his own experience seems to be at least as important as those, as we have already pointed out. However, Ganivet's use of this term in his *Idearium* seems to have taken it almost literally from the ideas expressed by Théodule Ribot in his book *Les maladies de la volonté* (2002). Ricardo Senabre showed it when he spoke of the presence in this work of "modified" passages from Ribot's book (Senabre 1974, 597). As a severe critic of Ganivet, José Ortega y Gasset also referred to it in an article published in 1908 in the following way:

> Ganivet—del cual tengo una opinión muy distinta de la del común entre los jóvenes, pero que me callo por no desentonar inútilmente—leyó un librito, muy malo por cierto, de Th. Ribot, a la moda entonces, se entusiasmó y soltó la especie de la *abulia* española. Ahora bien; de *abulia* no cabe hablar sino cuando se ha demostrado la normalidad de las funciones representativas. Un pueblo que no es inteligente, no tiene ocasión de ser abúlico. Sin ideas precisas, no hay voliciones recias. (Ortega 1946, 113)

> Ganivet—of whom I have a very different opinion from that of the common among young people, but which I keep silent for not being uselessly out of tune—read a little book, very bad indeed, by Th. Ribot, fashionable then, he got excited and released the species of the Spanish apathy. However; we cannot speak of aboulia except when the normality of the representative functions has been demonstrated. A people that is not intelligent, has no occasion to be lazy. Without precise ideas, there are no strong volitions. (Ortega 1946, 113)

An example of this aboulia is found in sexuality. In the case of Schopenhauer, it shows a marked misogyny as a result of the consideration that this phenomenon was something intrinsic to the human being, but should be transcended. The only way to transcend this passionate will is asceticism. For Schopenhauer, the satisfaction of pleasure generated such a hole that led to boredom; therefore, to avoid this situation, the only way was to have so much will that one manages to control one's own body. We are, therefore, before a frankly suggestive paradox that, in my opinion, is also manifested in Ganivet. Both authors are aware of the importance of the will in the human being, but they perceive the disadvantages that it has for humanity itself.

> Dígase lo que se quiera, todo requiere un fin en el mundo, y el gran desencanto llega cuando en el fin más alto se descubre el vacío. Un amor sin objeto es muy bonito, pero muy poco consistente; un amor con objeto es más prosaico, más duradero y embrutecedor en demasía; porque ese objeto es la cría de los hijos, en los cuales no sólo está la finalidad del padre, sino que tampoco puede estar la suya propia. Así, todo lo que el hombre crea tiene fines aparentes que se alejan como el horizonte visible; el horizonte está en los ojos y no en la realidad, y nuestro fin, que es cooperar a una obra inacabable, aunque tenga un valor real, es inapreciable y hasta digno de desprecio. (Ganivet 1943, II, 1030)

> Say what you want, everything requires an end in the world, and the great disappointment comes when the highest end is discovered emptiness. A love without an object is very beautiful, but very inconsistent; a love with an object is more

prosaic, more enduring and too brutalizing; because that object is the rearing of the children, in which not only is the father's purpose, but also his own can not be. Thus, everything that man creates has apparent ends that recede like the visible horizon; the horizon is in the eyes and not in reality, and our goal, which is to cooperate with an endless work, even if it has real value, is priceless and even worthy of contempt. (Ganivet 1943, II, 1030)

Ganivet shows that the will is related to the primitive phenomenon of the human. In fact, he concludes that the natural state is that of "permanent fornication" (Ganivet 1943, II, 1031), a really direct phrase with which it tries to show the human will to live. Now, it uses precisely this direct terminology and whose connotation is negative to insert the degeneration or social decay of which we have previously spoken. The will, therefore, can be decadent if it falls into uncontrolled primitivism. In turn, its opposite, apathy, is also a symptom of illness.

WILL AND DESIRE

Persons with enough will to have the maximum control over themselves approach a kind of trans-subjectivity and manage to free themselves from the chains of nature due to their own ideas and spirit. What we have just indicated can be clearly seen in the work *The Sculptor of His Soul*. This complex work shows the complex and conflicting mind of its author. In it, the vicissitudes of a sculptor, Pedro Martir, who pretends to be free, are narrated. That is, exercising will through the overcoming of a series of obstacles: faith, first, love, and last, death. The character represents this search for a volitional element that transcends subjectivity. At the end of the day, Ganivet shows once again the rejection of the nature of the body and its drives (something typical of the moment), although—as we saw before—he gives great importance to the psyche which, on the other hand, is inserted in a body. Schopenhauer (2014) also affirmed something similar when he said that existence was fatigue and work. So when a limited mind (in Schopenhauer's words) rested, boredom took place. This is the result of when the brain becomes a parasite or pensioner; an aspect that, on the other hand, María Zambrano (2011) also defended.

In this sense, Ganivet in his *El escultor de su alma* writes:

Desprecia ese cuerpo inerte, / que es el nido de tu muerte! / Ése es el caos, donde yace / luz que en tu muerte nace. (Ganivet 1943, 743)

Despise that inert body, / which is the nest of your death! / That is chaos, where lies / the light that is born in your death. (Ganivet 1943, 743)

The volition aims to break with nature in a Platonic ideal of liberation from corporeal wishes, which are the basis of illness, and to move toward a contemplative determination—one of Ganivetian obsessions—to activity—another of the key concepts of his thought.[7]

Death in Ganivet's work is a projection, a desire that goes beyond the merely rational. This moment becomes the only way to overcome the limitations of nature and the body. Furthermore, the Spanish writer and thinker accepts certain aspects of rationalism, although once again he transcends the merely rational. In this sense, we can consider Ganivet to be in a permanent search for the trans-subjective. Hence, it would not be enough to speak of solipsism[8] or an orientalist (nirvanic) perspective of the Andalusian's work. Death, petrification, is a mechanism to blur the limits of reality and its potential ability to affirm the spirit and overcome the slag of the body (de la Fuente Ballesteros 2010).

The idea-force[9] of petrification is interesting as a saving mechanism for the spirit. In the story *Las ruinas de Granada* (The Ruins of Granada), Ganivet tells us how a wise man and a poet visit the ruins of a city devastated by the eruption of magma from a volcano. In this story, the poet interprets the volcano itself as a kind of sculptor who has managed to generate "another form of life." In it, the human being is not necessary since the idea of the city lives in the air (Ganivet 1943, II, 712). Again that liberating trans-subjectivity. A thanatophilic trans-subjectivity in which the numeral seems to be above the phenomenal. In this sense, the positivism that we saw in Ganivet with his somewhat medicalized vision of the world (phenomenon) also coexists with a liberating human understanding. For this reason, the human being can also be conceived as a creative force that seeks to go beyond what has not yet happened.

Once some of the elements of Ganivet's work have been seen, it is time to return to his *Idearium español* (Spanish Idearum) to explain the ideal where the writer's homeland is based. If his ideal man in Greece is Ulises, indicates the Andalusian, for Spain it is Don Quixote. This point again leads us to the baroque link that Ganivet makes explicit. At the end if we remember the prudent self-control that Baltasar Gracián raised, we could consider that there are certain concomitances with the idea of Ganivetian petrification. Now Ganivet is much more tragic than the baroque thinker. Yo morrirée cuando quiera (I will die whenever I want), he writes, desperate for being "too much in the world" and tied up with a limiting rope, "como esclavo a la especie" (as slave to the species).

Ganivet is therefore a paradoxical writer and emergent thinker as few others are. His work reveals the conflict of the time and the concern for health degradation so present at that time. Now, he is a disbelieving writer since, for him, life has no purpose and therefore it is necessary to transcend it. In addition, although he advocates action and the will to save Spain, he is also aware that excess action is what caused the problems of this.

Porque no creo ni en el real ni en el aparente; no amo la acción ni la contemplación, ni me encanta el misticismo ese convencional de los que después de una buena comida se elevan a las alturas para hacer una digestión espiritual. Cuando se es cínico hay que vivir en el tonel, como Diógenes, y cuando se es escéptico hay que dejarse atropellar por el tren que viene resoplando y morir creyendo que el tren es una ficción, y cuando se es cristiano hay que serlo como san Francisco de Asís. Estos ejemplos son los que vivifican las doctrinas, pues, aunque el hecho práctico destruya realmente la doctrina, ésta queda en pie, a pesar de los fracasos y hasta en virtud de ellos. Porque lo que afirma a la idea no es la demostración práctica . . . sino la convicción personal. Si en el momento supremo Jesús se hubiese acobardado, y por medio de una hábil rectificación se hubiera librado de la cruz, toda la generosa moral evangélica valdría hoy lo que un episodio de *La Ilíada*. (Ganivet 1943, II, 1025–26)

Because I don't believe in the real or the apparent; I do not love action or contemplation, nor do I love the conventional mysticism of those who after a good meal rise to the heights to make a spiritual digestion. When you are cynical you have to live in the barrel, like Diogenes, and when you are skeptical you have to let yourself be run over by the train that comes puffing and die believing that the train is a fiction, and when you are Christian you have to be like Saint Francis of Assisi. These examples are those that vivify the doctrines, because, although the practical fact really destroys the doctrine, it remains standing, despite the failures and even by virtue of them. Because what affirms the idea is not the practical demonstration . . . but the personal conviction. If in the supreme moment Jesus had cowed, and by means of a skilful rectification he had got rid of the cross, all the generous evangelical morals would be worth today what an episode of The Iliad would be worth. (Ganivet 1943, II, 1025–26)

Again, what the Granada-born writer puts on the table is his voluntarism, but also his lack of faith and his desire to overcome the contingency, the body. But we must not be mistaken; the theme of the action in our writer is connected with a worldview in which reality is presented as fragmentary and disaggregated, which depends on the subjectivity of the issuer, compared to the apparent objectivity of the Zolian novel. It is not about painting the world, representing it, but about promoting the representation of the subject. Again, Zambrano (2011) comes to mind when he stated that the human being represents himself as his own need and exemplified this statement by recalling the work of Benito Pérez Galdón. Moreover, Unamuno in his work does not stop giving us his idea of the world, of its representation. Let us remember what he says in "El sentimiento trágico de la vida" (The tragic feeling of life), "Yo soy el centro de mi universo, el centro del universo" (I am the center of my universe, the center of the universe; Unamuno 1968, VII, 136). This is not an exceptional case, since Remy de Gourmont in *Sixtine: roman de la vie cérébrale* makes his hero say: "Le monde, c'est moi, il me doit la'existence, je l'ai creé avec mes sens et il est mon slave et nul sur lui n'a de pouvoir" (1890, 13) (The world is me, it owes me existence, I created it with my senses and it is my slave and no one has power over it).

All this can be verified in his fictional characters, such as Pío Cid. This supposes the victory of the authentic man (interior) in front of everything external, the affirmation of the will in front of the society. The action of the protagonist of *Los trabajos del infatigable creador Pío Cid* (The works of the indefatigable creator Pío Cid) is passive, since it is not carried out through direct actions, but through ideas (de la Fuente Ballesteros 2013). Nordau did not know the Ganivetian proposals, but his diagnosis would have been similar to the one he makes about other artists: he is aboulic, he abhors activity, he would be, therefore, a degenerate, a disciple of Schopenhauer with his philosophy of renunciation (asceticism), who he does not adapt to the circumstances, without forgetting that he can be branded as egotistical—we can find all this in the first part, in chapter 3, entitled "Diagnosis." In the same way, the pathographies carried out on Ganivet years later were no less compassionate, spurred by the suicide of the writer, since the opinion of a contemporary doctor has been spoken of "progressive general paralysis caused by syphilis" to, in years closer to us, "schizoid personality" (Conde Gargollo 1964, 60), "fasothymic psychosis" (Marín de Burgos 1982, 126), "schizo-epilepsy" (Rojas Ballesteros 1985, 134), or simply "cyclical depression" (Castilla del Pino 1965). That is to say, a hermeneutical tradition that repeats a turn of the century cliché where the maintenance of certain prejudices of the medical discourse can be observed, where the artist continues in the nebula of the detour.

NOTES

1. Max Simon Südfeld, known as Max Nordau (1849–1923), was a Jewish Hungarian writer who wrote in German. He was promoter of Zionism and became paradigmatic representative of positivism. Among his works are *The Conventional Lies of Civilization* (1883), *Paradoxes* (1885), and his great success, *Degeneración* (1892). He pilloried writers and artists of the time, whom he medicalized and analyzed as clinical cases. Not symbolists, like Rimbaud, or naturalists, like Zola, escaped a diagnosis that puts their anomaly on the table.

2. The work was translated into English and the following year, in 1894, the French version appeared. The Spanish version was translated by Nicolás Salmerón in 1902.

3. The arguments are repeated over and over again in these writers, as in the case of the novels by Díaz Rodríguez (de la Fuente Ballesteros 2001–2003), and in the

treatment given to the "Babylonian" Lutecia, source of all evils, the great city of vice and decadence, an example of progress, but also of degeneration (from Fuente Ballesteros 2014), as can be seen in the first part of *Entartung* of Nordau.

4. In any case, we must remember how Unamuno starts from a certain confidence in progress that leads him to invoke the necessary Europeanization of Spain, until shortly after opting for the Spanization of Europe, with his claim to Don Quijote and his madness. Alberich analyzes Unamuno's speech from his proximity to positivism to his exhaustion and disillusionment with scientism; so that since 1898 we can read, in the interview with Azorín, this about material progress, which can only be useful if "liberating man from the anguish of daily bread and from a great number of human miseries, leaves him a place to look up and attend to their union with God" (Azorín 1999, 139). This article is in the line of *Meditations*, as Laureano Robles (1999) points out.

On the other hand, there are two articles by Unamuno published in La Nación de Buenos Aires entitled "Progressism and history" on August 8 and 15, 1920, where he emphasizes that the denial of progressivism is not the denial of science (Unamuno 1997).

5. Miguel de Unamuno, *La voluntad nacional* España, March 19, 1915, available in the Repositorio Documental de la Universidad de Salamanca.

6. Pardo Bazán, in modern French literature, pointed out the romantic affiliation of turn-of-the-century thought: "The hundred years of literature that I am going to review are of a very intense life, with rapid changes in taste and in the aesthetic ideal; But whoever comes with me to the end of the path will notice how, under the aspect of diversity and even opposition, the consequences of the same principle, the roots of the same tree, are hidden. From the first moment there existed in the new literature, so lush, so brilliant, the germ of decadence into which it has come to sink; and note that it is not the same to decline due to a congenital disease than to die at the right time, a natural death, having lived healthy. Certainly all literary forms are perishable; and yet (as in the individuals of the human race), their constitution and the balance of their health vary greatly. Thus, French classicism brought elements of normal life, while the period that begins in romanticism and now ends in disintegration and anarchy, has not been, in its painful magnificence, but the development of a morbid germ, a beautiful clinical case" (1911, 7–8). This has also been underlined by Praz and Carter, among others.

7. As Javier Herrero points out: "This superiority of contemplation over active life is essential to the man; that is, the highest operation of the human soul is the vision of the ideal world, and, especially, the contemplation of Supreme Love, of the Artificer. Active life is justified only when it pursues the realization of some ideal" (Herrero 1966, 281–83).

8. O ideas mother, concept that takes from the idea-force of Alfred Fouillé (Robles Egea 1997).

9. "Over time, one becomes convinced that there is too much in the world; that there are no proper ends of man, because the only ends (which are generation and conservation) are non-individual specific ends, that one does not do anything essential, or if one does something it is to engender another being analogous or worse, and that

all the others occupations are formal or imitative and like efflorescence produced by organic rubbing. We are neither more nor less than engines; we work to pull a weight, to produce movement, to give this or that useful result. But what is the engine itself? It seems like something because it can work on its own, because it gives off sparks or steam or smoke; but its reason for being is the machine. So we, to make the deceit more pleasant, we throw several things out and we believe that they are something, being that what is positive is the machine of our species, to which we are yoked as slaves" (Ganivet 1943, II, 1028–29).

REFERENCES

Alberich, J. "Unamuno y la duda sincera." *Revista de Literatura* XIV-27–28 (1958): 210–25.

Alonso, Luis Enrique. *La crisis de la ciudadanía laboral*. Barcelona: Anthropos, 2007.

Ardila, J. A. G. *Etnografía y politología del 98. Unamuno, Ganivet y Maeztu*. Madrid: Biblioteca Nueva, 2007.

Arjona, D. King. "La *voluntad* and *abulia* in Contemporary Spanish Ideology." *Revue Hispanique* 74 (1928): 573–671.

Aronna, Michel. "'Pueblos enfermos': The Discourse of Illness in the Turn-of-Century Spanish and Latin American National Essay." Doctoral thesis. Pittsburgh: University of Pittsburgh, 1993.

Azaña, Manuel "En torno a Ganivet." *La pluma* 9 (1921): 87–96.

Azorín. "Charivari en casa de Unamuno." In *Caras y más caras de 1900*, edited by M. P. Celma. Valladolid: Difácil, 1999: 137–41.

Balandier, George. *El Desorden. La Teoria del Caos y las Ciencias Sociales*. Barcelona: Gedisa, 1989.

Bataille, Georges. *La littérature et le mal*. París: Gallimart, 1957.

Baudelaire, Charles. *Salones y otros escritos sobre Arte*. Madrid: Visor, 1996.

Baudelaire, Charles. *Poesía completa. Escritos autobiográficos. Los paraísos artificiales. Crítica artística, literaria y musical*, edited by Javier del Prado and José A. Millán Alba. Madrid: Espasa-Calpe, 2000.

Bergua, José Ángel. *Patologías de la modernidad*. Madrid: Catarata, 2019.

Beriaín, Josetxo. *Modernidades en disputa*. Barcelona: Anthropos, 2005.

Berrios, G.E., and M. Gili. "Will and Its Disorders: A Conceptual History." *History of Psychiatry* 6, no. 21 (1995): 87–104.

Baroja, Pío. "Nieztsche y su Filosofía." *Revista Nueva* 1 (1899): 33–39.

Bauman, Zygmunt. *Modernidad y ambivalencia*. Second edition. Barcelona: Anthropos, 2011.

Campos Marín, Ricardo. "La sociedad enferma: Higiene y moral en España en la segunda mitad del siglo XIX y principios del XX." *Hispania* 55/3 (1995): 1093–112.

Campos Marín, Ricardo. *Alcoholismo, medicina y sociedad en España (1876, 1923)*. Madrid: CSIC, 1997.

Campos Marín, Ricardo. "Entre el vicio y la enfermedad. La construcción medico-social del alcoholismo como patología en España (siglos XIX y XX)." *Trastornos adictivos* I, no. 3 (1999): 280–86.

Canguilhem, Georges. *Lo normal y lo patológico*. Buenos Aires: Siglo XXI, 1971.

Cardwell, Richard. "*Los raros* de Rubén Darío y los médicos chiflados finiseculares." In *Rubén Darío y el arte de la prosa. Ensayo, retratos y alegorías*, edited by Cristóbal Cuevas, 55–77. Málaga: Publicaciones del Congreso de Literatura Española Contemporánea, 1998.

Carter, Alfred Edward. *The Idea of Decadence in French literatura, 1830–1900*. Toronto: University of Toronto Press, 1958.

Castilla del Pino, C. "Para una patografía de A. Ganivet." *Ínsula* 228–229 (1965): 5.

Cerezo Galán, Pedro. "Ángel Ganivet: el excéntrico nihilista de la modernidad." In *Ganivet y el 98*, edited by Antonio Gallego Morell and Antonio Sánchez Trigueros, 11–43. Granada: Universidad, 2000.

Conde Gargollo, E. "Angel Ganivet y su sentido histórico." *Cuadernos Hispanoamericanos* 172 (1964): 51–71.

Comín Comín, Francisco. *Historia económica mundial. De los orígenes a la actualidad*. Madrid: Alianza editorial, 2012.

Compagnon, Antoine. *Les antimodernes de Joseph de Maistre à Roland Barthes*. Paris: Folio, 2005.

Compagnon, Antoine. *Los antimodernos*. Barcelona: Acantilado, 2007.

Cordova, Abraham. "The Romantic Cenacle: An Intellectual Coterie in Search of Status." *European Journal of Sociology* 18–2 (1977): 335–55.

Díaz, Rodríguez. *Ídolos rotos*. Caracas: Monte Ávila, s.f., 1901.

Díaz, Rodríguez. *Camino de perfección, Apuntaciones para una biografía espiritual de Don Perfecto y varios ensayos* [1910]. Caracas: Ed. Cecilio Acosta, 1942.

Díaz, Rodríguez. Manuel. *Sangre patricia* [1902]. Caracas: Monte Ávila, 1972.

Durkheim, Emile. *De la division du travail social*. Second edition. París: PUF, 1991.

Ehrenreich B. *Una historia de la alegría*. Barcelona: Paidós, 2008.

Földényi, László *Melancholy*. New Haven: Yale University Press, 2016.

Foucault, Michel. *Los anormales*. Madrid: Akal, 2001.

Foucault, Michel. *El nacimiento de la clínica. Una arqueología de la mirada médica*. Madrid: Siglo XXI, 2007.

Fuente Ballesteros, Ricardo de la. "Ganivet y Schopenhauer: pensadores intempestivos." In *Anales de Literatura Española* 12 (1996), serie monográfica 2, *Shopenhauer y la creación literaria en España*, edited by de M A. Lozano, 89–100.

Fuente Ballesteros, Ricardo de la. "Patología y Regeneración: en torno al héroe ganivetiano." *Siglo diecinueve* 4 (1998): 75–91.

Fuente Ballesteros, Ricardo de la. "Mundo fenoménico/mundo nouménico: una clave finisecular (Unamuno/ Ganivet/Baroja)." *Ottawa Hispanic Studies* 24 (1999): 245–60.

Fuente Ballesteros, Ricardo de la. "Manuel Díaz Rodríguez y el viaje a París." *La nueva literatura hispánica* 5–7 (2001–2003): 47–59.

Fuente Ballesteros, Ricardo de la. "El artista enfermo. El caso Darío." *Siglo Diecinueve* 7 (2001): 147–60.

Fuente Ballesteros, Ricardo de la. "Enfermedades y vacunas en Gómez Carrillo." In *El cuerpo enfermo: representación e imágenes de la enfermedad*, edited by Ricardo de la Fuente Ballesteros and Jesús Pérez Magallón, 85–96. Valladolid: Universitas Castellae, 2007.

Fuente Ballesteros, Ricardo de la. "Tanatología ganivetiana." *Anales de Literatura Española Contemporánea* 35, no. 1 (2010): 287311.

Fuente Ballesteros, Ricardo de la. "Enfermedad y escritura: el caso de Ángel Ganivet." In *Literatura y locura*, edited by Andreas Kurz, 137–57. Madrid, Guanajuato: Universidad de Guanajuato, 2012.

Fuente Ballesteros, Ricardo de la. "Paradigma heroico y pasividad." In *Perfiles del heroísmo en la literatura hispánica de entresiglos XIX-XX*, edited by Luis Álvarez Castro and Denise DuPont, 173–90. Valladolid: Edit. Verdelís, 2013.

Fuente Ballesteros, Ricardo de la. "Las sensaciones parisinas de Gómez Carrillo." *Siglo diecinueve* 20 (2014): 287–303.

Fuente Ballesteros, Ricardo de la. "El fin de siglo y sus resistencias frente al progreso: Díaz Rodríguez." In *Numancia: representaciones culturales de la resistencia en el mundo hispánico*, edited by Ricardo de la Fuente Ballesteros and Vicente Pérez de León, 21–36. Madrid: Wisteria, 2019.

Ganivet, Ángel. *El escultor de su alma y otros textos dramáticos*. Valladolid: Universitas Castellae, Ediciones Críticas *Siglo diecinueve*, 2000.

Ganivet, Ángel. *Obras completas*. Madrid: Aguilar, 1943.

Ganivet, Ángel. *España filosófica contemporánea y otros ensayos*. Madrid: Librería Beltrán, 1930.

Ganivet, Ángel. *Idearium español y El porvenir de España*. Granada: Tip. Lit. Vda. e Hijos de Sabate, 1897.

González Serrano, Urbano. *La sociología científica*. Madrid: Librería de Fernando Fe, 1884.

Gourmont, Remy de. *Sixtine: roman de la vie cérébrale*. París: A. Savine, 1890.

Gutiérrez Nájera, Manuel. "El arte y el materialismo." In *El modernismo visto por los modernistas*, edited by Ricardo Gullón. Barcelona: Labor, 1980.

Herman, Arthur. *La idea de decadencia en la historia occidental*. Santiago de Chile: Editorial Andrés Bello, 1998.

Herrero, Javier. *Ángel Ganivet: un iluminado*. Madrid: Gredos, 1966.

Huertas García-Alejo, Rafael. *Locura y degeneración. Psiquiatría y sociedad en el positivismo francés*. Madrid: Consejo Superior de Investigaciones Científicas, 1987.

Iglesias de Ussel, Julio. "Ángel Ganivet en la sociología del siglo XIX." In *Conocimiento y realidad. Estudios en homenaje a Jorge Riezu Martínez*, edited by José Antonio Portero Molina, 271–94. Salamanca: Edit. San Esteban, 2004.

Jurkevich, Gayana. "Abulia, Nineteenth-Century Psychology, and Generation of 1898." *Hispanic Review* 60 (1992): 181–94.

Kupperman, Karen O. "Apathy and Death in Early Jamestown." *The Journal of American History* 66, no. 1 (1979): 24–40.

Láscaris, C. "El pensamiento filosófico de Ángel Ganivet." *Revista de la Universidad de Buenos Aires* 22 (1952): 453–533.

Lorry, Anne-Charles. *De melancholia et morbis melancholicis.* Paris: Cavelier, 1765.

Marín de Burgos, J. *Patografía de Ganivet.* Madrid: Pirámide, 1982.

Mead, George H. *Espíritu, persona y sociedad.* Barcelona: Paidós, 1982.

Nordau, Max. *Degeneración.* Madrid: Librería de Fernando Fe, 1902.

Nye, Robert A. *Crime, Madness and Politics in Modern France. The Medical Concept of Nacional Decline,* Princeton, NJ: Princeton University Press, 1984.

Ortega y Gasset, José. "Algunas notas." In *Obras completas.* Volume I. Madrid: Revista de Occidente, 1946.

Pardo Bazán, Emilia. *Literatura francesa moderna. Obras completas de Emilia Pardo Bazán.* Volume 37. Madrid: V. Prieto y Cía, 1911.

Pick, Daniel. *Volti delle degenerazione. Una sindrome europea 1848–1918.* Florencia: La Nuova Italia Editrice, 1999.

Pine, Richard. *The Dandy and the Herald.* London: Palgrave Macmillan, 1988.

Praz, Mario. *La carne, la muerte y el diablo en la literatura romántica.* Barcelona: El Acantilado, 1999.

Ramsden, Herbert. *Ángel Ganivet's Idearium español. A Critical Study.* Manchester: University Press, 1967.

Ramsden, Herbert. *The 1898 Movement in Spain. Towards a Reinterpretation with Special Reference to "En torno al casticismo" and "Idearium español."* Manchester: University Press, 1974.

Ribot, Théodule. *Les maladies de la volonté.* Paris: L'Harmattan, 2002.

Robles, Laureano. "El mal del siglo (texto inédito de Unamuno)." *Cuadernos de la Cátedra de Miguel de Unamuno* 34 (1999): 99–131.

Robles Egea, Antonio. "El neoidealismo y la rebelión de Ángel Ganivet contra el positivismo: sobre Alfred Fouillée y la teoría de las ideas." *RILCE* 13, no. 2 (1997): 201–21.

Roche Cárcel, Juan Antonio. *La sociedad evanescente.* Barcelona: Anthropos, 2009.

Rojas Ballesteros, L. *El atardecer de Ángel Ganivet.* Granada: Caja Provincial, 1985.

Schopenhauer, Arthur. *Parerga y Paralipómena I.* Madrid: Trotta, 2014.

Senabre, Ricardo. "Ganivet y el diagnóstico de la abulia." In *Studia Hispanica in Honorem R. Lapesa,* 595–99. Madrid: Gredos, 1974.

Shaw, Donald L. *La Generación del 98.* Seventh edition. Madrid: Cátedra, 1997, 45–70.

Soldevilla Pérez, Carlos. *Ser barroco. Una hermenéutica de la cultura.* Madrid: Biblioteca Nueva, 2013.

Santibáñez Tió, Nil. *Ángel Ganivet, escritor modernista.* Madrid: Gredos, 1994.

Trigo, Benigno Luis. "Enfermedad y escritura: el impacto de la decadencia y de la degeneración en la obra de cuatro escritores hispanoamericanos." Doctoral thesis, Yale University, 1992.

Trigo, Benigno Luis. *Ensayos.* Madrid: Publicaciones de la Residencia de Estudiantes, 1916–1918.

Trigo, Benigno Luis. *El sentimiento trágico de la vida. Obras Completas.* VII. Edited by Manuel García Blanco. Madrid: Escelicer, 1968.

Trigo, Benigno Luis. *Artículos en "La Nación" de Buenos Aires (1919–1924).* Edited by Luis Urrutia Salaverri. Salamanca: Universidad de Salamanca, 1994.

Unamuno, Miguel. *Andanzas y visiones españolas*. Madrid: Renacimiento, 1929.

Unamuno, Miguel. *Obras Completas*. vol. VII, Madrid: Escelicer, 1968.

Unamuno, Miguel. *De patriotismo espiritual. Artículos en "La Nación" de Buenos Aires 1901–1914*. Ed. and notes of Víctor Ourimette. Salamanca: Ediciones Universidad de Salamanca, 1997.

Zambrano, María. *Notas de un método*. Madrid: Tecnos, 2011.

Chapter Three

The Language of a Sick Nation

Epidemics and Environmental Destruction in the Narratives of Lima Barreto

Zélia M. Bora

Epidemics and global pandemics are not novelties to the human spirit. In the Southern Hemisphere, especially in Latin America, epidemics and pandemics inaugurated colonial governance. During the sixteenth century, Spanish conquistadors carried smallpox, measles, typhus, mumps, and other contagious diseases to present-day Mexico, Ecuador, and Peru. These diseases devastated indigenous civilizations in the New World. Later, North America, the Pacific Islands, Australia, and New Zealand were also locations that "experienced similar populations decline following European colonization in the 18th and 19th centuries" (Harvard Library n.d.). In the specific case of Brazil, the process of modernization was unfavorable to the most vulnerable sectors of society. When endemic diseases spread, most of the victims were poor individuals. The relationship between epidemics, modernization, and nature's destruction is a relevant interrelationship to understand the social complexities of Brazilian modernization.

Thousand narratives were written about Brazilian modernization, especially if one considers the press and literary production. Daily journalism and literature were at first the basic genres that registered the paradoxes of the process. No other writer in the beginning of the twentieth century deserves more attention than Lima Barreto. Not only because of the variety of genres he chose to represent these realities, but because he faithfully portrayed the historical marginalization of subaltern classes.

By demonstrating their social dilemmas as well as their painful economic integration within society, Lima Barreto's journalism was very supportive of class struggle.

In the present discussion, I will explore the relationship between the nation and illness in his masterpiece *Triste Fim de Policarpo Quaresma* (Sad End of Policarpo Quaresma). His critique inaugurated an intellectual tradition that anticipated discussions on national identity, otherness inequalities, and social justice. Although he did not participate in the organization of the First Week of Modern Art (1922) that launched the Brazilian literary "Modernismo," Lima Barreto's writings demonstrate the paradoxes of Brazilian modernity and his disillusionment with the republican political project. Labeled as a pré-moderno (pre-modern) writer by the traditional Brazilian critic Alfredo Bosi (1936–2021) in his "Historia Concisa da Literatura Brasileira," Lima Barreto's work is better comprehended under the light of the term modernity. Judging by his work, he became one of the first critics of modernity in Latin America. Although Lima Barreto was not contrary to progress, he demonstrated that modernity had a paradoxical side that was not beneficial to all citizens. In other words, the Brazilian project of modernity was problematic and biased. He understood it and was entirely conscious about his intellectual role as a critic of modernity, especially its paradoxes. Taking into considerations his writings, it is evident that the historical moment he lived in was underlined by a series of epidemics. Nevertheless, the life of Lima Barreto was not too different than many Brazilians that had to face inequality, poverty, racism, and illness, including the madness of his father as well as his own health problems. The same question regarding the nation's paradoxes posed to the protagonist of *Triste Fim de Policarpo Quaresma* is also posed to the reader. The question, O que é a Pátria (What is the Nation?), is overemphasized throughout the novel. If the same question could be asked to the writer, the answer would be probably that the nation was ill because of the real and symbolic illnesses, such was the threat of the fragile democratic order after the establishment of the republic. The nation was affected by numerous epidemics that affected at that time, Rio the Janeiro. Besides, Brazil was also ill because of the corruption of its republican leaders.

As the capital of the empire, Rio de Janeiro in the beginning of the twentieth century not only gained the reputation of a "modern" city but also of a place where infectious diseases followed each other in quick succession. Like other colonial outposts, the spread of epidemics accompanied the history of Brazil throughout the end of nineteenth century and the beginning of the twentieth century.

The existence of a cycle of contagious diseases also defined the politics of modernization of Rio de Janeiro (capital of Brazil from 1763 to 1960). Earlier transplanted liberalism (through positivism) emphasized the guidelines of the republic and its own path to modernization. Based on French, British, and other "civilized nations," the project had two complementary steps to reach modernity. First by architecture, second by science specially medicine,[1] and third, "progress through positivism" (see Merquior 1982). All of them were part of the urgent necessity to transform the country into "a modern nation."

By establishing a "new" postcolonial order under new representations, architecture and medicine became the backbone of Brazilian modernity. Both were implemented at the same time. Metaphors related to the words old and new were constantly used to differentiate the past from the present, the rich from the poor. There was not in the strict sense a project of urbanization. The old was systematically destroyed to give place to the new. Most of the time, they had to coexist side by side. The pronounced destruction of "Morro do Castelo" in 1905 was one of these controversial projects. It did not only destroy the entire hill together with its biomass but also human dwellings. In his "O Subterrâneo do Morro do Castelo" (The Underground of Castle Hill), Lima Barreto considered it "um insano trabalho" (an act of madness) perpetrated by politicians.[2] The environmental impact of the gradual destruction of Morro do Castelo was devastating since the colonial times. In 1811, there was a flood in which several people died (Barros 2002, 10). But the environmental impact did not count. Progress could not wait. The natural environment of Rio is unique to Brazilian environment. Surrounded by five islands and hills, the urban idyllic vision was one of the most beautiful in the world. Nevertheless, its beauty was altered by the process of colonization and later modernization. The destruction of Morro do Castelo (The Castle Hill), previous named "São Januário," Descanso, and finally Castelo, became a paradigm of how nature was altered according to human interest. Its destruction turned Rio into an environment conducive to the spread of pathogens. In the sixteenth century, The Castle Hill was chosen by the Portuguese to be a fortress against French invasions. In order to avoid "foreigner" occupations of the hill, the Portuguese founded the city of São Sebastião. (Barros 2002, 11). The geographical composition of the hill was characterized by the presence of ponds, swamps, and mangroves. Gradually, the lagoons were dissected, the swamps and mangroves drained, and embankments were made over the sea. Thus, tunnels were constructed and the hill was gradually destroyed to build avenues. Besides the ecological impact, the hill's destruction impacted thousands of human lives (Barros 2002).

EPIDEMIC RIO, EPIDEMIC NATION—A
HISTORICAL CONTEXTUALIZATION

In order to understand the relationship between modernity and illness in the Brazilian context and how Lima Barreto developed his critical outlook, it is necessary to go back to the last decades of nineteenth-century Rio. The precarious social integration of former slaves and freed Blacks into society was very stricken. Between 1850 to 1860, they were the predominant inhabitants of the "cortiços" (favelas). Initially inhabited by free Blacks and later by emancipated slaves, the "cortiços" were located in the center of Rio de Janeiro. On January 26, 1893, a remarkable fact took place in the "cortiço" Cabeça de Porco (Pig head). Their inhabitants woke up to an eviction order from all the houses. The dwellings were collective, and the number of the inhabitants was estimated around two thousand people. Although the population resisted the removal and the loss of their belongings in the pouring rain, they were allowed to go up the hills. The "spontaneous" transference of the poor population to the hills of Rio was the origin of the "favelas" (shanty towns of Rio) (Chalhoub 2006, 21). Later, soldiers who came back from War of Canudos[3] (1897), poor Portuguese immigrants, and other individuals went to live in those places. Like the "cortiços," the favelas were considered a place of "dangerous classes." The increasing number of the favelas each year represented how the socially disabled were outside the benefits of progress. Considered as a place "averse" to order, the favelas became places of poverty, brutality, and death. Although social dynamics helped some individuals reach certain social mobility, most of the populations remained in the lower stratum. In general, racism as well as social class differences prevailed as a social practice that made it almost impossible for the first poor republican generation to stand upward. Regarding the inhabitants of the "cortiços," they were not considered dangerous only because they were poor but because they also "represented components of resistance." Their removal was also considered an effort to "disarticulate collective memories associated to social urban movements" (Chalhoub 2006, 25).

The policies of Brazilian modernization systematically included popular as well as scientific racist ideas current in Europe in the nineteenth century to explain society (see Dezem 2011). They were proclaimed by certain members of the elite classes. These ideas were used first to justify slavery and later were incorporated in the permanent political imaginary. Thus, a "tropical" version of social Darwinism and scientific racism became social "reminders" to implement the division between desirable and non-desirable citizens. Regarding the environment where the poor lived, it was considered not only dangerous but also degrading and unhealthy. In 1850, after the spread of yellow fever and cholera, a campaign of destruction of "unhealthy" dwellings as well as natural sites was initiated. These outbreaks gave origin to a cycle of epidemics that remained active throughout the Old Republic (1889–1930). Among them were yellow fever, tuberculosis, malaria, and smallpox. In this way, the timid social reforms of the empire became the political and social agenda of the republic. Left to their own devices without material conditions to ascend to the benefits offered by modernity, the excluded populations were not only seen as dangerous classes but "they also offered danger of contagion" (Chalhoub 2006, 29). The height of tension between the poor and the ruling classes occurred in the so-called vaccine revolt (1904). At that time, Lima Barreto was twenty-three years old and extended his sympathy toward the protesters by writing.

LIVING AND WRITING MADNESS

Besides fatal pathogens that affected individuals, mental disorders in general were simply called madness. They affected many Brazilians between the end of nineteenth century and the twentieth century. The incidence during slavery and after it called the attention of one of the most prominent Brazilian psychiatrists, Juliano Moreira (Fry 2000; Levine 1971). He innovated the treatment of mental illness in Brazil. He believed that the causes of insanity were basically social and not defined by the race of the patient. He was also against the confinement of the patients and humanized their treatment the best as his could (Nardi, Carta, and Shorter 2021). Lima Barreto had problems with alcohol and because of this, he was taken twice to the psychiatric house. The experience was written in "O Cemitério dos Vivos" (1919–1920) (Cemetery of the Living).

No other writer has better represented the relationship between modernity, environmental destruction, epidemics, madness, and inequality in Brazilian society like Lima Barreto. Born in Rio de Janeiro (1881–1922), Afonso Henriques de Lima Barreto was a man of his time, but still very current in the present context we are living (post-pandemic society). There is a substantial difference between the madness of Lima Barreto and his character Policarpo Quaresma, object of my analysis.

In the novel *Triste Fim de Policarpo Quaresma*, the main actions are basically around the rise and the fall of its protagonist, Policarpo Quaresma. As a middle-class man and intellectual, he lived in a mixed neighborhood with affluent and less affluent inhabitants. Despite the fact that Quaresma lived in a small farm in the suburb, the streets were always crowded by the "spontaneous" growth of the modern city. According to the narrator,

Os subúrbios do Rio de Janeiro são a mais curiosa cousa em matéria de edifica-
ção da cidade. Nada mais irregular, mais caprichoso, mais sem plano qualquer,
pode ser imaginado. (Barreto 2008, 70)

The suburbs of Rio de Janeiro are the most curious thing in terms of building
the city. Nothing more irregular, more capricious, more without any plan, can
be imagined.

Like other modern streets, different individuals of different social classes
circulated:

Há pelas ruas damas elegantes, com sedas e brocados, evitando a custo a
lama ou o pó lhe empanem o brilho do vestido; há operários de tamancos; há
peralvilhos à última moda; há mulheres de chita; e assim pela tarde, quando essa
gente volta do trabalho ou do passeio, a mescla se faz numa mesma rua, num
quarteirão, e quase sempre o mais bem posto não é o que entra da melhor casa.
(Barreto 2008, 74)

There are elegant ladies in the streets, wearing silks and brocades, struggling to
avoid the mud or dust that tarnishes the shine of their dress; there are clog workers; there are dandies in the latest fashion; there are calico women; and so in
the afternoon, when these people come back from work or from a walk, the mix
takes place on the same street, in a block, and almost always the best dressed is
not the one that comes from the best house.

Very rich in details, the imagery of the neighborhood underlines the social
class differences among the individuals. In this sense, the difference between
silk and calico worn by the women reinforces these differences. These differences seem deeper when the narrator shows the uncontested and precarious
situation of the Blacks in general and the poor. Poverty and lack of education
made the poor neighborhoods more susceptible to contagion. The narrator
uses the metaphorical word "courtship" to make reference to the easy and
"natural" possibility of contagion:

Além disto, os subúrbios têm mais aspectos interessantes, sem falar no namoro
epidêmico e no espiritismo endêmico; as casas de cômodos (quem as suporia
lá!) constituem um deles bem inédito. Casas que mal dariam para uma pequena
família, são divididas, subdivididas, subdivididas, e os minúsculos aposentos
assim obtidos, alugados à população miserável da cidade. Aí, nesses caixotins
humanos, é que se encontra a fauna em menos observada de nossa vida, sobre a
qual a miséria paira com um rigor londrino. (Barreto 2008, 72)

Besides, the suburbs have more interesting aspects, not to mention epidemic
courtship and endemic spiritualism; rooming houses (who would have thought

of them there!) are one of them quite unheard of. Houses that would barely fit a small family are divided, subdivided, subdivided, and the tiny rooms thus obtained are rented out to the miserable population of the city. It is there, in these human coffins, that the least observed fauna of our lives is found, over which misery hovers with a London rigor.

By 1904, besides yellow fever, bubonic plague, and tuberculosis, smallpox was recurrent. On November 10, a protest related to the public health broke out. Apparently, the immediate cause for this was the mandatory vaccination. Nevertheless, according to the historians Nicolau Sevecenko and José Murilo de Carvalho (Carvalho 1987; Sevecenko 2018), the public was discontent with the politics of the republic. Despite the violent repression of the police, the crowd was not intimidated. They did not disperse and were in the streets for five days. Lima Barreto stayed at home but did not fail to express his solidarity to the protest. He was twenty-three years old and registered it in his first novel (metaphorically represented by a shoes revolt; Gruner n.d.). The vaccine revolt, as it was named, was also mentioned in his *Intimate Diary* published posthumously. Writing about the incident, Lima Barreto wrote:

Essa mazorca teve grandes vantagens 1 demonstrar que o Rio de Janeiro pode ter opinião e defende-la com armas na mão. 2. Diminuir um pouco o fetichismo da farda 3. Desmoralizar a Escola Militar. Pela primeira vez, eu vi entre nós não se ter medo de homem fardado. O povo, como os astecas no tempo de Cortez, se convenceu de que eles eram mortais. (1953, 1222)

This provocateur had great advantages: 1 demonstrating that Rio de Janeiro can have an opinion and defend it with weapons in hand. 2. To reduce a little the fetishism of the uniform 3. To demoralize the Military School. For the first time I saw among us not to be afraid of man in uniform. The people, like the Aztecs in Cortez's time, became convinced that they were mortal.

In his *Diário Íntimo*, he distinguishes the police targets very well. Most of them belonged to "dangerous classes." Many died; others were hurt and deported. At the same time, smallpox was taking its victims. In 1904, there were thirty-five hundred dead and eighteen hundred admissions to the hospital. The numbers given by the Centro Cultural da Saúde (Cultural Health Center) is doubtful. It says that 945 were arrested and only thirty died (Dandara 2022). Historians estimate a higher number, including deported individuals. The narrative of Lima Barreto did not estimate numbers but emphasized the facts and the violence against the civil population, especially the poor.

Eis a narrativa do que se fez no sítio de 1904. A polícia arrepanhava a torto e a direita pessoas que encontrava na rua. Recolhia-as às delegacias, depois juntavam na Polícia Central, aí violentamente, humilhantemente, arrebatava-lhes os cós das calças e as empurrava num grande pátio. Juntadas que fossem algumas dezenas, remetia-as à ilha das cobras onde eram surradas desaprecia. Eis o que foi o terror do Alves; o do Floriano; o do Floriano foi vermelho, o de Prudente, branco, e o de Alves, incolor, ou antes de tronco e bacalhau. (Barreto 1953, 1223)

Here is the narrative of what was done at the state-of-siege in 1904. The police rounded up people they found on the street randomly. After this, they took them to the police stations, then gathered them in the Central Police, there violently, humiliatingly, he snatched the waistbands of their pants and pushed them into a large courtyard. As many as a few dozen, he would send them to the island of snakes where they were beaten down. This is what Alves' terror was; Floriano's; was red, Prudente's white, and Alves' colorless, or rather tie & whipping.[4]

Contrary to Lima Barreto, his character Policarco Quaresma lacks critical outlook toward the nation. His tendency to emotional and fanatical feelings prevents him from a reasonable criticism of the republican policy. It is very possible that Lima Barreto wanted to distinguish the difference between the country, territory, and the nation. Quaresma's nationalism at first is "static" and particularizes only the territory. His "naïve" nationalism first embraces the cultural traditions of Brazil (Barreto 1953, 21), the nature, and its romantic literature to mention just a few (Barreto 1953, 29). His conflicting ideas between his perspective and with what was really going on absorbs his entire existence. Not only he has particular opinions about Brazil but also lives according to his personal judgment, without confronting reality. His neighbors think he is "um homem esquisito e misantropo" (weird and misanthropic) but harmless. He works for the Brazilian government. His colleagues do not understand his intellectual efforts "to feed" this "strange" nationalism. Despite his singularity, Quaresma is always polite and respects others. Like Dom Quixote, he is to some extent an idealist. Immersed in his own meditations, Quaresma one day writes a requirement to the National Congress to change the official language of Brazil. Although the Portuguese spoken in Brazil is different from the Portuguese spoken in Portugal, Quaresma intends to substitute it for Tupi-Guarani, an indigenous language that was not spoken by the majority of the population. Despite the lexical contribution of the language to Brazilian Portuguese, the plea sounded in the beginning of the twentieth century exotic and absurd. He also disregards the fact that not only Portuguese is spoken in Brazil but also other indigenous languages besides Tupi-Guarani. By doing this, he proclaims the essentialism of one language over the other. In fact, Tupi-Guarani was spoken and taught in Brazil during the eighteenth century. Later, it was forbidden by the Marquis of Pombal in order to sabotage the Jesuit project and permanence in Brazil to continue the pedagogic colonization of native Brazilians. The argumentation of Quaresma, however, did not include this historical support and his project sounded absurd to all of his friends. As a result, Quaresma was not only openly exposed but became a target of national mockery. His friends and acquaintances had the same opinion: he was mad. Slowly, madness got in the way of the common sense.

In the absence of "a common sense," Quaresma decides to surrender himself to the care of his own land. But a strange encounter with a colony of ants in his kitchen launches a new challenge to the "hero." The ants not only attacked his grains for planting but also stung him. Quaresma devotion to agriculture gradually made him aware of the society that surrounded him that he never perceived:

> De resto, a situação geral que o cercava, aquela miséria da população campestre que nunca suspeitara, aquele abandono de terras à improdutividade, encaminhavam sua alma de patriota meditativo a preocupações angustiosas. (Barreto 2008, 94)

> Moreover, the general situation that surrounded him, that misery of the rural population that he had never suspected, that abandonment of land to unproductivity, led his meditative patriot's soul to anguished concerns.

Suddenly, Quaresma's unrequited love for the nation turned into flurry of questions centered on the land to make it productive. By selling its fruits, he started thinking the land could be profitable. The profit from the sales of an enormous quantity of avocado was ridiculous while the financial efforts to reach the market were absurd (Barreto 2008, 95). Not giving up, Quaresma thought about selling his corn. To his dismay, the plantation had been totally destroyed by the ants. Not only the corn but also his orange trees. Gradually, he also became aware of the bureaucratic difficulties to selling his products. Despite that, Quaresma understanding of society was still uncritical.

By showing complementary images that suggest the reader that the worse still was about to come to the hero, the narrator shows that malady is a persistent component in the lives of the poor inhabitants around Quaresma's resort that he never noticed before:

> Pelos seus olhos passaram num instante aquelas faces amareladas e chupadas que se encostavam nos portais das vendas preguiçosamente; viu também aquelas crianças maltrapilhas e sujas, d'olhos baixos, a esmolar disfarçadamente pelas estradas; viu aquelas terras abandonadas, improdutivas, entregues às ervas e insetos daninhos; viu ainda o desespero de Felizardo, homem bom, ativo e trabalhador, sem ânimo de plantar um grão de milho em casa e bebendo todo o dinheiro que passava. (Barreto 2008, 100)

In an instant, those yellowed, sunken cheeks that lazily leaned against the sales
portals passed through his eyes; he also saw those ragged and dirty children,
with their eyes downcast, begging surreptitiously on the roads; he saw those
abandoned, unproductive lands, given over to weeds and harmful insects; he
also saw the despair of Felizardo, a good, active and hardworking man, not in
the mood to plant a grain of corn at home and drinking all the money that earned.

Besides the loss of the orange trees and the corn, an epidemic also decimated
the turkeys, chickens, and ducks (Barreto 2008, 100). He also was fined for
not paying the taxes on his products. Even though disgrace was knocking at
his door, he still could not be critical enough. His idea of public administration was oversimplified and personified. To him, the leader was the system,
and the system was the leader. There is no accusation or criticism on the narrator side against him, although Quaresma in the end explains his deeds as an
act of love to the country and his self-deception could save him.

> ele como muitos homens honestos e sinceros do tempo, foram tomados pelo
> entusiasmo contagioso que Floriano conseguira despertar. Pensava na grande
> obra que o Destino reservara àquela figura plácida e triste, na reforma radical
> que ele ia levar ao organismo aniquilado da pátria, que o major se habituara a
> crer a mais rica do mundo, embora, de uns tempos para cá, já tivesse dúvidas a
> certos respeitos. (Barreto 2008, 115)

> he, like many honest and sincere men of the time, was seized by the contagious
> enthusiasm that Floriano had managed to arouse. He thought of the great work
> that Fate had reserved for that placid and sad figure, of the radical reform he was
> going to bring to the annihilated organism of the homeland, which the major had
> grown used to believing as the richest in the world, although, for some time now,
> he had already doubts in certain respects.

But the most bizarre attitude related to Quaresma "deranged" insights was
expressed through his support to the destruction of the democratic order.
He surprises the reader for engaging himself into a political action in an
army coup. Later, this irreversible act causes him a feeling of deep disap-
pointment and self-politic deception, but it will be too late to recuperate the
past. "Unable" to be critical, he gradually becomes a tragic hero who builds
his own downfall while he plunges in to the world of regrets. However,
the complexity of his "solitaire madness" had its flirtations with authority
personified by Marshall Floriano Peixoto. Nicknamed Marechal de Ferro
(Iron Marshal), he was the first dictator of Brazil. Ironically, the madness of
Quaresma is expressed through his nationalism. His punishment is to be sent
with other volunteers to a headquarters located in an old "cortiço" destroyed
by its anti-hygienic environment. As a prison officer, old and tired of his

fruitless actions, he thinks about his death. Suggesting he lived a life of misunderstanding, the narrator reveals to the reader Quaresma's most complete self-confession:

> Iria morrer, quem sabe naquela noite mesmo? E que tinha ele feito de sua vida? Nada. Levara toda ela atrás da miragem de estudar a pátria, por amá-la e querê-la muito, no intuito de contribuir para sua felicidade e prosperidade. Gastara sua mocidade nisso, a sua virilidade também; e agora que estava na velhice, como ela o recompensava, como ela o premiava, como ela o condecorava? Matando-o. E o que não deixara de ver, de gozar, de fruir, na sua vida? Tudo. (Barreto 2008, 151–52)

> He was going to die, who knows, that very night? And what had he done with his life? Anything. He had taken all of her after the mirage of studying the country, for loving it and wanting it very much, in order to contribute to its happiness and prosperity. He had spent his youth on it, his manhood too; and now that he was old, how did she reward him, how did she reward him, how did she honor him? killing him. And what had he not stopped seeing, enjoying, enjoying in his life? All.

Even though the narrator shows sympathy to Quaresma, he also shows that the fruits of his actions are irreversible and cannot be extinguished by his will. Quaresma lost his youth, his friends, his farm (which was consumed by the ants, plagues, and insects), and his entire life daydreaming. His example suggests the reader that dreams and illusions are overcome under the light of truth. And the past cannot be recuperated.

CONCLUSION

Writing in a period of urban turmoil in which the country was struggling to leave behind the old and proclaim modernity, Lima Barreto was not only a witness but also a critic of modernity. Some literary critics classify, inadvertently, his literature as a pre-modern literature; however, a careful look at the politics of modernization that came with the advent of the republic exemplifies that Lima Barreto was skeptical with the project of modernization. A hundred years later, his work is still an unquestionable testimony on the history of Brazilians' attempt to insert the country into modernity. Published in 1915, *Triste Fim de Policarpo Quaresma* is considered his masterpiece. The novel is marked by his undeniable taste for irony. As an aesthetic device with the satiric fillings around Quaresma, the writer suggests that we must be always attentive to political seductions and avoid mistakes that can make our lives worse. Quaresma's pathetic existential condition was less harmful when he dedicated himself to his monotonous daily activities. plowing the land from which he expected in vain "the fruits." But Quaresma's sin was to have a deceitful vision about society and specifically about the republic. Like other protagonists, like Clara dos Anjos and Isaías Caminha, he will be consumed by a deviant society composed by dishonest, unscrupulous individuals and a government that failed to providing the basis to a fairer society. Beyond Clara dos Anjos and Isaías Caminha, the unhappy saga of Policarpo Quaresma portrays the saga of a nation composed by thousands of naïve individuals that like Mr. Quaresma maintain unrealistic and ingenuous beliefs in the republic. His naivety prevents him from seeing the many evils of the nation, and his blind faith encapsulates the writer's sad smile of his own non-conformist social outlooks. Thus, the authorial narrator foresees Quaresma's ultimate deception by the epigraph in the beginning of the narrative. To Quaresma and Lima Barreto, the obstacles created by the social web were too deep and unfair. But unlike Quaresma, Lima Barreto was a critical antagonist of the nationalist excesses until his death in 1922. To him, the nation was literally and symbolically ill. This statement is also present in between the lines of *Triste Fim de Policarpo Quaresma*. In the end of his novel, the protagonist was overpowered by madness and old age. Nevertheless, the madness of Quaresma was symbolic quixotic. Like Dom Quixote, Quaresma is a tragic hero who comes to terms with his own madness at the end of his life. Quaresma regrets his past deeds and resumed his acritical love for the nation. To Lima Barreto, madness was a social condition that affected him and his father. His madness was loaded by the anguishes of his daily existence that included the systematic racism that transformed him into a collateral victim among several in Brazilian society.

NOTES

1. According to Nisia Trindade Lima, in her article "Public Health and Social Ideas in Modern Brazil" (2007), public health in Brazil achieved remarkable development at the turn of the twentieth century thanks in part to physicians and social thinkers who made it central to their proposal for "modernizing" the country. Public health was more than a set of medical and technical measures; it was fundamental to the project of nation building. Regarding the adoption of tropical medicine, it is evident that it collided with the so-called popular medicine used by the population (in general related to indigenous and African cultures). European or Western medicine was accepted by physicians "who faithfully (and passively) reproduced European medicine in their mainly tropical countries. Brazil's concerted efforts after the turn of the century to sanitize cities and backlands can be seen as evidence of how closely governments and medical authorities adhered to the highly successful methods used

to eradicate disease in European colonies and the U.S. South." See Peard (1997). As I tried to demonstrate, in Rio the vaccine became highly politicized.

2. O Subterrâneo do Morro do Castelo, Correio da Manhã, 1905.

3. In general, the common citizen did not trust the government. The War of Canudos was not entirely forgotten (1896–1897) at that time. The settlement was destroyed and the survivors killed.

4. Here Lima Barreto makes an allusion to slavery and the present by mentioning the punishment inflicted to the poor caught during the riot. It is also important to emphasize that they were arrested independently, whether they participated in the rebellion or not.

REFERENCES

Barreto, Lima. *Prosa Seleta*. Volume Único. Editora Nova Aguilar. 2008.

Barros, Paulo Cezar de. "Onde nasceu a cidade do Rio de Janeiro?(um pouco da história do Morro do Castelo)." *Revista geo-paisagem* 1, no. 2 (2002): 1–19.

Brown University Library. "Positivism." *Brazil Five Centuries of Change.*, n.d. https://library.brown.edu/create/fivecenturiesofchange/chapters/chapter-4/positivism/

Carvalho, Jose Murilo. *Os Bestializados: O Rio de Janeiro e a República que não foi.* São Paulo: Companhia das Letras, 1987.

Chalhoub, Sidney. *Cidade Febril: Cortiços e Epidemias na Corte Imperial.* São Paulo: Companhia das Letras, 2006.

Dandara, Luana. "Cinco Dias de Fúria: Revolta da Vacina envolveu muito mais do que a insatisfação com a vacinação" *Portal Fio Cruz* (2002). https://portal.fiocruz.br/noticia/cinco-dias-de-furia-revolta-da-vacina-envolveu-muito-mais-do-que-insatisfacao-com-vacinacao

Dezem, Rogério Akiti. "The Brazillian Belle Époque." *Academia.edu*, 2011. https://www.academia.edu/1302231/_The_Brazilian_Belle_%C3%89poque_new_ideas_old_paradigms

Fry, Peter. "Politics Nationality and the Meanings of 'Race' in Brazil." *Daedalus* 129, no. 2 (2000): 83–118.

Gruner, Clóvis. "Metáforas da revolta: impressões e representações da Revolta da Vacina em Lima Barreto." n.d. http://www.snh2011.anpuh.org/resources/anpuhpr/anais/ixencontro/comunicacao-coordenada/dialogos%20impertinentes%20historia%20arte%20e%20literatura/ClovisGruner.htm

Harvard Library. "Contagion Historical Views of Diseases and Epidemics." Curiosity Collections, n.d. https://curiosity.lib.harvard.edu/contagion/feature/colonialism-and-international-medicine

Leonardo, Lucas. "O Jovem Lima Barreto e a Hegemonia Positivista." *Roteiros Literários*, 2020. https://medium.com/roteirosliterarios/o-jovem-lima-barreto-e-a-hegemonia-positivista-cb3fa2207bfc

Levine, R. "Some Views on Race and Immigration during the Old Republic." *The Americas* 74, no. S1: 373–80.

Lima, Nísia Trindade. "Public Health and Social Ideas in Modern Brazil." *American Journal of Public Health* 97, no. 7 (2007): 1168–77.

Merquior, J.G. "More Order than Progress? The Politics of Brazilian Positivism." *Government and Opposition* 17, 4 (1982): 454–68.

Nardi, Antonio E., Mauro G. Carta, and Edward Shorter. "The Remarkable Juliano Moreira (1872–1933): An Afro-Brazilian Psychiatrist, Scientist and Humanist in an Environment of Slavery and Racism" *Brazilian Journal of Psychiatry* 43, no. 3 (2021): 237–39.

Peard, Julyan G. "Tropical Disorders and the Forging of a Brazilian Medical Identity, 1860–1890." *Hispanic American Historical Review* 77, no. 1 (1997): 1–44.

Sevecenko, Nicolau. *A Revolta da Vacina. Mentes Insanas, Corpos Rebeldes.* São Paulo: Editora Unesp, 2018.

PART II

Chapter Four

Guatemalan Expressions

*Memorials and Private Reflective
Spaces during the Internal Conflict
and COVID-19 Pandemic*

Martha C. Galván-Mandujano

In Guatemala, many abuses have been committed against the Mayan indigenous people; they have suffered racism, displacement, dispossession of land, and lack of access to resources. Many massacres and abuses happened during the internal conflict that led to a genocide. Throughout the civil war, the highest number of killings were between 1981 and 1983—the genocidal period known as La Violencia. The most affected areas experiencing widespread killings, torture, and rape were in the Department of Quiché, particularly in the mountainous Ixil and the Ixcán regions. As part of the peace process ending Guatemala's thirty-six years of armed internal conflict, the 1996 Oslo Accord for Firm and Lasting Peace established the Commission for Historical Clarification (CEH). The CEH's mandate was to explain why both the government and the guerrillas committed extreme acts of violence. According to the report of the CEH, of the total 626 villages where massacres occurred, 344 were registered in the Quiché region alone. In "Guatemala Memory of Silence," the CEH reported that the Guatemalan Army was responsible for 93 percent of the atrocities and massacres committed against Mayan indigenous victims (CEH 1999, 42). Moreover, many of the victims died of illnesses and hunger when they escaped to the highlands. At present, Mayan communities continue to fight for the rights to their ancestral lands; many communities have been evacuated in agrarian conflicts. In addition, they are struggling with an increase of COVID-19 cases; in the past three years, they have not received as much assistance from the government due to the lack of educational resources in their native languages and medical aid reaching the remote areas.

   This study aims to provide an overview of the mechanisms and factors that have influenced the creation of spaces to represent the struggles of various Maya Achí indigenous communities in Baja Verapaz, represented by memorials and murals in cemeteries. The historical background, forced disappearances, and displacement of many Maya Achí allows analyzing the different levels of systematic discrimination against this group during the conflict, post-conflict and during the COVID-19 pandemic. Moreover, the pandemic has affected these communities: there has been an increase in coronavirus cases because of lessened health education campaigns and prevention efforts. Finally, the chapter explains how the memorialization processes and the educative work both about the internal conflict and the COVID-19 pandemic come mainly from non-governmental organizations and international organizations, not the state.

STRUGGLE AND MASSACRES DURING THE INTERNAL CONFLICT IN RABINAL AND THE AGRARIAN CONFLICTS DURING COVID-19 IN COMMUNITIES OF BAJA VERAPAZ

The rural community of Rabinal is one of eight municipalities and dozens of villages in the Department of Baja Verapaz and the historic hub of the Maya Achí. The violence against the indigenous communities became a reality for this area beginning in the early 1980s. Even though this municipality was not a combat zone throughout the internal armed conflict, it did not escape the violence associated with the government's scorched-earth campaign. The army considered this area to be of strategic importance because of its geographical location as a corridor from Guatemala City to the Alta Verapaz and the Ixcán, Quiché (Rothenberg 2012, 70). Rabinal also began to experience the state-wide increase in political repression of selective violence in late 1979 that targeted community leaders and land activists (Museo Comunitario Rabinal Achí [MCRA] 2003).

   The massacres were also positioned between two of Guatemala's genocidal regimes—that of President Fernando Romeo Lucas García (1978–1982) and General Efraín Ríos Montt (1982–1983). Between 1981 and 1982, the Lucas García regime initiated a counterinsurgency campaign that massively repressed indigenous communities under the guise of destroying the social base of the guerrillas. As part of this strategy, the regime began the establishment of the civilian defense patrollers that consisted primarily of local indigenous men and boys who the army pressed into patrolling villages to seek out guerrillas. Many were compelled to become members and commit atrocities and participate in massacres out of fear and that their non-participation would be seen as evidence of sympathizing with the guerrillas (Stewart 2008, 236). At this time, the systematic massacres of indigenous villages began in earnest. On March 23, 1982, a military triumvirate led by Ríos Montt took power from Lucas García in a coup d'état to preserve the military's hold on power. Throughout his seventeen-month tenure, Montt continued the massacres initiated by his predecessor but in a more systematic manner, and his regime led one of the most brutal campaigns against the indigenous communities during the entire armed internal conflict. Alongside the massacres, the scorched-earth campaign against the communities included the intentional destruction and burning of their property, which included homes, tools, domestic animals, seeds, and harvests. The immediate effect of this material loss subjected survivors to hunger, illnesses, and exposure, forcing many to flee their villages and creating both internally displaced and refugee populations. In addition, this material loss had far-reaching effects for future generations as it destroyed traditional systems of inheritance and, consequently, the continuity of the community. The demolition of material culture also destroyed the sense of the individual self because this loss shattered the means by which the individual and the community as a group relate to one another (Dupuis 2005, 7). As the Recovery of Historical Memory Project report indicated, the assault on the community also destroyed social customs disrupting marriages as well as women's sense of identity associated with wearing traditional dress and its relation to a women's personal dignity (Proyecto Interdiocesano Recuperación de la Memoria Histórica [Guatemala], Catholic Institute for International Relations, and Latin America Bureau 1999, 44–49). The graphic drawings on several of the cemetery memorials in Rabinal capture this material loss and stand as visual reminders of the state's attempted eradication of their cultural identity for those who come to commemorate the dead. The CEH identified the Maya Achí of Rabinal as one of five Mayan groups against which the Guatemalan state committed "acts of genocide" (CEH 1999, 41).

Association for the Integral Development of the Victims of Violence in the Verapaces (ADIVIMA) was the first organization that began the initial memorialization efforts in Rabinal. The founding members of the association, comprised of the widows and survivors of massacres and human rights abuses in the early 1980s, date ADIVIMA's founding to April 24, 1994. This day marked the public burial of the remains of the seventy women and 107 children from the March 13, 1982, Rio Negro massacre, who were finally laid to rest following their exhumation (ADIVIMA n.d.). The members' activism grew out of their earlier association, the Widows and Orphans Committee, the forerunner to ADIVIMA, originally formed to exhume and publicly bury their relatives and build a monument in their memory (Stewart 2008, 237). With the financial support of national groups such as the National Coordination of Widows of Guatemala (CONAVIGUA) and other domestic and international human rights organizations, in November 1993, the Guatemalan Forensic Anthropology Team exhumed the remains of the March 13, 1982, massacred women and children who were buried in a clandestine grave (Stewart 2004, 266). In April 1994, the community held a public reburial and erected a small monument dedicated to the Rio Negro martyrs with the inscription "who gave their life for peace, whose blood fertilizes our land and represents the seed of truth, justice and hope" (Stewart 2004, 266). As the first public burial and monument of its type in the country, it attracted national media attention along with the attendance of Rigoberta Menchú; however, as Stewart notes, within two weeks the monument was destroyed with many suspecting that the military was responsible because of the proximity of the cemetery to the military base in Rabinal (Stewart 2004, 266).

As their mission expanded, the Widows and Orphans Committee became ADIVIMA to reflect their extended work to address poverty and other socio-economic issues. Their memorialization endeavors continue and focus on establishing memorials to preserve the memory of victims, continuing exhumations of clandestine graves, and ensuring proper burials. Indigenous women in Rabinal are at the forefront of these efforts, and they began to "break their silence" and "make known" the violence their communities suffered even as the armed internal conflict was ongoing (Doiron 2007, 85). In 1999, ADIVIMA succeeded in establishing the Museo Comunitario de la Memoria Histórica in Rabinal as the first historical memory museum in Guatemala that would address the impact of the civil war on the local Achí community. In their recovery of history memory, the museum reports that in the municipality of Rabinal, indigenous women were the most impacted by the internal armed conflict (MCRA 2003). In their memorialization work, their standpoint is grounded on their Achí identity and what was lost during the internal armed conflict. In general, not only did women witness the destruction of their communities, as symbols of the family, they were deliberately targeted with sexual violence and systematic rape during massacres aimed at destroying the seed (Doiron 2010, 80). Soldiers used their motherhood against them by using their children as instruments of psychological torture. The death of children threatens the lineage of families and entire communities. Pregnant women were particularly vulnerable to brutal methods of torture (MCRA 2003). Women who survived were more often widows who faced an uncertain economic, socio-cultural, and psychological future. Those with children faced additional challenges of supporting their children. Widows found their traditional gender roles upended, and many women attempted to work in the fields, taking on the traditional male role of tilling the soil. Others migrated to find jobs in a domestic labor market mainly in

Guatemala City, while others left their community to find work elsewhere and even join associations such as CONAVIGUA.

The Mayan people of Baja Verapaz, Guatemala, have struggled not only in the internal conflict. In the present, land activists have been killed and indigenous people evacuated from their lands. The agrarian conflicts were happening and continued during the pandemic. According to Peace Brigades International (PBI) in Guatemala, in April 2020 in the worse part of the pandemic, families denounced publicly that they were being forced to evacuated; private entities (landowners and private companies) were forcing them. The government and other international entities were not able to help. Washington, a community in Baja Verapaz comprising seventy families that has been forced to work since the nineteenth century for landowners (finqueros), was evacuated. PBI Guatemala stated that

> the families from the community of Washington lived now in the municipalities of Purhulá y Salamá with family members and friends. Now that they have been evacuated, they have difficulties surviving, since their crops were ubicated in the lands they lived was their means of subsistence. Even though the national organization Unit for the Protection of Human Rights Defenders in Guatemala (UDEFEGUA) and el Bufete Juríco de Rabinal (The Law Firm of Rabinal), have supported them with food. In the context of the pandemic, they live in economic, social, and psychological vulnerability. Many indigenous from various departments of Guatemala faced similar agrarian conflicts before and during the pandemic. (PBI Guatemala 2021)

In 2021 the Secretary of Agrarian Affairs, the institution that could try to solve agrarian conflicts, was shut down (PBI Guatemala 2021), leaving these communities displaced.

During the pandemic, many Achí Mayans were affected again economically due to travel restrictions, bringing memories of struggle from the internal conflict, because they could not go to Guatemala City because of government mandates. They relied on aid from organizations such as ADIVIMA and CONAVIGUA. In 2020 and 2021, these non-governmental organizations provided food assistance with the international help of organizations such as Trócaire, an agency of the Irish Catholic Church.

COVID-19 PANDEMIC BACKGROUND IN GUATEMALA

Guatemala confirmed the first case of coronavirus on March 13, 2020. The Guatemalan government declared a state of emergency in early March 2020, closing the national border, suspending unessential activities, banning interdepartmental travel (Guatemala is divided in departments/states), creating sanitary perimeters, and instituting a curfew (6 pm–4 pm) (Webb and Cuj 2020, 103). The pandemic left many Mayans economically and medically at a disadvantage. Many had been commuting to Guatemala City to work, sell their products in the informal economy, or receive medical assistance unrelated to COVID-19, such as cancer, dialysis, etc. Mayan communities had already been living in a permanent state of precarity before COVID-19; now they were facing additional challenges as the public crisis unfolded (Webb and Cuj 2020, 103). Also, the different restrictions and curfews brought memories of past trauma during the internal conflict because members of the army came to rural areas to reinforce the restrictions. PBI described in their bulletin of December 2021:

> People from communities in various regions of the country accompanied by PBI have described how the states of siege and curfews have had an extreme impact on the elderly population, as they have revived the memory of trauma experienced during the Internal Armed Conflict: "for those of us who lived through the war, it awakens that fear again. People were more afraid of the curfew than of the disease." (PBI 2021)

The government did not provide as much information, food, and medical assistance to the remote areas and indigenous communities at beginning of the pandemic. Cesar Armando Bol Chocooj wrote, "A loan of 450 million dollars from international organizations was urgently approved by the Congress. Very little of this money was directed to health. Beyond this, there are no specific emergency response plans that benefit the most vulnerable, including the Indigenous Peoples" (2020). Furthermore, the Guatemalan Congress granted special permission to the industrial business sector and protected state salaries. Still, most of the Guatemalan population participating in the informal economy did not receive the same aid (Bol Chocooj 2020). Another disadvantage for the indigenous community was the dissemination of information for prevention and vaccination campaigns. Many do not speak Spanish and did not have access to the internet and radio. The international community and government could not translate all the materials into their native languages. There are twenty-two Mayan languages (Instituto Nacional de Estadística 2018). The Maya Achí in the Baja Verapaz Department alone has 121,340 Achí native speakers and only a small group of Spanish speakers. Many flyers, documents, or radio announcements were only in Spanish and just a few indigenous languages and sometimes not in the Mayan vernacular language (Webb and Cuj 2000, 105). Even though the government awarded some international loans to help during the coronavirus crisis, the indigenous communities did not receive much aid. Part of the aid to prevent the spread of the coronavirus was "to order the Academy of Mayan Languages to translate some informational materials about the coronavirus into the country's Indigenous languages, and distribute them through the media, above all in social media" (Bol Chocooj 2020). Nevertheless, the materials were limited. Unfortunately, some of the communities do not have internet or television, and some of them do not have radio signals or batteries for radios. Another problem is that they barely have electricity, if at all (Bol Chocooj 2020).

The increase of COVID-19 cases brought more instability to these rural and Mayan indigenous communities. The World Health Organization recorded that from January 3, 2020, to July 15, 2022, a total of 963,117 COVID-19 cases were confirmed in Guatemala with 18,756 deaths. In July 2022, there was a wave of new cases; in a period of twenty-four hours, 7,747 cases were confirmed on July 15, 2022 (World Health Organization n.d.). By August 23, 2022, the cases increased to 1,085,456 and deaths to 19,352. The Area of Baja Verapaz estimated 833 confirmed cases ("Tablero COVID-19 Guatemala" 2023). The country currently has classified sixty-six municipalities of Guatemala in red, 224 in orange, fifty in yellow, and none of them in green, worrying many of the municipalities. Most of the rural areas, including communities in Baja Verapaz, were classified as red and orange ("Tablero de COVID-19" 2023, 33).

ADIVIMA's member Mario Sical stated that they provided food, prevention kits, and information for prevention (communication with author, July 14, 2022). Feliciana Macario Tevalan, a member of CONAVIGUA, explained in a message that many of the information about COVID-19 was made via radio, but as explained some communities do not have radio signal or access (communication with author, July 14, 2022). They also taught indigenous members how to reinforce their immune system using traditional herbal medicines.

FUNCTION OF MEMORIALS

In general, genocide memorials serve multiple purposes. These include honoring the memory of victims, serving as symbolic forms of reparations, acting as sites of healing, bearing witness, and aiding in truth and justice initiatives. In the case of recent COVID-19 deaths, many cemeteries' spaces have been assigned only for these deaths. I broadly define memorials to include monuments, murals from the internal conflict, murals for COVID-19 awareness and honoring, cemeteries, spaces for COVID-19 deaths in cemeteries, and private reflective spaces associated with remembrance, memorialization, and to teach about the pandemics. Louis Bickford (2014) notes that leading the efforts to build memorials that expose the crimes of the state are civil society groups representing victims who demand a voice in writing their collective narrative. Thus the memorials analyzed in this chapter provide a collective narrative expressed in private and public spaces during the internal conflict and recent COVID-19 pandemic.

I situate these sites and activities in a relational context prescribed by Bickford depending on the goals of any memorial—whether they serve a private/reflective function or public/educative role, and whether they are located on authentic or symbolic sites. This is especially important when I viewed private reflective sites within cemetery walls and other private memorials spaces. Within these spaces, I approached my understanding of these memorials as both observer in a space that was not intended for outside, let alone foreign viewers, and as witnesses to atrocities. In looking at Mayan women's experiences, I searched for women's names on cemetery markers, chapel crosses, and memorial plaques that listed massacre victims specially from Baja Verapaz. In addition, I examined if any of the memorials depict their lives post-genocide/post-conflict and the impact on their roles as women given the social disintegration caused by the conflict. While the genocidal period spans the period between 1981 and 1983, known as La Violencia, as I mentioned before. The armed internal conflict continued for another thirteen years. On the other hand, this department continues to struggle with the pandemic and agrarian conflicts.

FUNCTION OF PRIVATE REFLECTIVE SITES AND CEMETERIES

This chapter investigates memorials located within cemeteries and private reflective spaces and present areas assigned for COVID-19 deaths. In this context, I trace the early efforts at memorialization which began as part of the attempt to fight for the exhumation of massacre victims and the rights of those displaced by the internal armed conflict as well as to prosecute war criminals. Predominate in this effort has been organizations such as ADIVIMA. Their work is confined to the geographic region of the Verapaces. ADIVIMA funded the first memorialization efforts in Rabinal and included the construction of massacre memorials. Most of them located in the public cemetery/Cementerio General de Rabinal, which contains ten memorials that commemorate massacres against the Achí Maya community.

Many of the victims who were exhumed, identified, and reinterred dwell within the space of private reflective memorials that function as places for survivors and communities to heal, commemorate, mourn, honor, and remember. Whether this space takes the form of a commemorative grave in a public cemetery, a memorial altar, or even a clandestine grave, private reflective sites are often "victim-driven projects" that originate at the local level (Bickford 2014, 504). As locally driven memorials, they represent both the universal suffering of the Mayan people as well as atrocities felt by specific Mayan communities who experienced La Violencia; those killed were in the majority Maya. Additionally, the violence these communities sustained in the early 1980s as part of the army's counterinsurgency strategy was the worst in terms of the destruction of Mayan life and culture since the Spanish conquest five hundred years prior (Garrard-Burnett 2015, 182). While there are untold numbers of clandestine graves and other private reflective sites throughout the zones of conflict, I particularly focus on the Cementerio General in Rabinal, which has become one of the most important sites of expressions of memorialization in Baja Verapaz, Guatemala.

As Victoria Sanford notes (2003, 17), cemeteries are "sacred places" in which the rituals associated with burial and mourning are public acts and the remains of the dead are entombed in accordance with community funeral rites. Yet many of the memorials throughout the Baja and Alta Verapaces commemorating the victims of massacres exhumed from clandestine graves and reinterred in a public burial space portray scenes of violent deaths that are out of harmony with Maya spirituality. Although exhumations form part of "re-dignifying" victims (Henderson, Nolin, and Peccerelli 2014, 98), the rituals of reburial do not necessarily bring closure, especially if justice has eluded these communities (Garrard-Burnett 2015, 182). Even though many of the remains of victims have been identified and reinterred, it does not replace the Maya Achí rituals of death that would have brought complete closure to loved ones and the entire community had death occurred as part of the natural life cycle. Something similar happened with COVID-19 deaths, in the article "Nadie puede llorar a las víctimas de la pandemia/Nobody can cry for the victims of the pandemic" (Menchú 2021), bodies were buried without a name in the national cemeteries. One of the images from Oliver de Ros explains, "En la sección de Covid-19 del Cementerio *La Verbena*, la mayoría de los fallecidos son anónimos, y para los familiars resulta muy difícil poder encontrar a sus seres queridos/In the section of COVID-19 of La Verbena's Cemetery, the majority of the deceased are anonymous, and for the family members is difficult to find them" (Menchú 2021). Another image shows gloves left behind, not markers identifying the deceased. Sometimes families paid people in charge of the cemeteries to put a cross or flowers, trusting that the tomb was assigned to the corresponding family member (Menchú 2021).

On the other hand, during the internal conflict, massacre victims whose bodies were often mutilated and discarded in clandestine graves disrupted the harmonious relationship between the living and the dead, thereby upending the cultural bonds of the communities. For those victims not buried in clandestine graves, the army's counterinsurgency tactics that included the total destruction of communities left behind mutilated and desecrated corpses among the ruins of devastated villages. Fear often hindered survivors from returning to their communities to reclaim the dead as the army banned surviving families from burying relatives and, if they did usually return days later, they found victims devoured by animals and decomposing (Rothenberg 2012, 48–49). This type of systematic destruction not only physically attacked communities, but it also assaulted the cultural life of the communities, especially the spiritual elements of Mayan life. Dupuis (2005, 8) reports on the physical and psychological damage on the mental health of unfinished mourning on the Plan de Sánchez community who were not able to complete the mourning process until after the exhumations were completed in 1994—a full twelve years after the massacre. She notes that the "farewell death ritual" is an essential part of Maya Achí culture (Dupuis 2005, 8). This ritual establishes a new type of harmonious relationship between the living and the dead that allows the dead to look after the well-being of the living, especially through dreams in which deceased relatives convey messages and advice. In turn, the living ensure the dead rest in peace by holding the farewell ritual and inter the dead in a sacred place where the living can come to pray, leave flowers and candles, and commemorate. It is not possible to maintain this relationship if survivors have not recovered the remains of the dead and laid them to rest in a place where they can be honored by the living (Garrard-Burnett 2015, 186). Unless properly buried, the souls of the deceased inhabit in a "liminal space" in which they dwell between earth and their final resting place (Green 1994, 245). Moreover, as La Violencia intensified, it became difficult to hold traditional funerals out of fear of holding large gatherings and the inability to obtain funeral necessities such as coffins, food, and incense (Zur 1998, 202). The disruption of the death ritual placed particular hardships on widows who had to suppress expressions of grief if they were unable to perform funerary rituals, especially if there was uncertainty over the whereabouts of their spouse's remains. Emotional and physical suffering manifested itself on women's bodies in the form of illnesses among those who experienced dreams and apparitions of unburied husbands and fathers whose bodies have not been located or given a proper burial (Zur 1998, 224; Garrard-Burnett 2015, 186). While not a visual feature of the cemetery memorials, the emotional and physical trauma that women experienced caused by funeral disruptions is a noteworthy visual element in many of the murals I discuss later. Furthermore, mourning for a person who died violently and establishing the next level of relationship with the dead is difficult and not fully realized until the remains are identified and the dead accorded their proper status (Garrard-Barrett 2015, 186). Exhumations became an important political tool in the hands of widows because the exhumed sites refute the official government narrative that their family members were guerrillas, given that no weapons were found among the victims' remains in mass graves and many were blindfolded and bound. This material evidence grants the victims a form of silent testimony that contributes to the historical narrative that a genocide did occur amid a political climate in which the generals continue to refute this claim. In the highlands of Guatemala, the public cemetery in Rabinal contains the reinterred remains of hundreds of massacre victims of the genocidal scorched-earth policy of the late 1970s and early 1980s.

ANALYSIS OF THE CEMENTERIO GENERAL IN RABINAL

Entering the Cementerio General in Rabinal that houses the remains of massacre victims feels intensely personal. Upon arrival, one is the witness of the active movement or visitation of family members to this space. Before entering this private reflective space, I encounter the community through a series of banners that wrap the outside walls that summarize various themes pertaining to the history and culture of the Achí people. One series defines their history as one of struggle and resistance that is captioned above an area map that directs attention to the location of the massacres that occurred in Pichec, Agua Fría, Río Negro, Panacal, Plan de Sánchez, Xesiguian, and Chicupac. Accompanying this narrative are the headshot photos, names, and, in some, images the ages of the massacre victims who are presented underneath a heading that reads "these are the faces of our families, friends, neighbors massacred during the armed internal conflict, all of them had dreams, a longing, a life" (my own translation and photo taken from banner in Rabinal, June 2017). (See figure 4.1.)

This banner series also provides specific maps of Plan de Sánchez, Panacal, and Pichec that diagrams each community and the location of dwellings as they existed prior to the massacres. (Photograph taken on my visit to Rabinal in June 2017). (See figure 4.2.)

Another section of the exterior wall displays a memory collection of photographs representing the cultural life of the Maya Achí—an initiative of the Association for Justice and Reconciliation, an organization founded by survivors to demand accountability and justice. The photos exclusively feature women engaged in a range of communal activities from the spiritual to the artisanal. Accompanying this series of photos is a cursive script that simply but powerfully lists a range of human rights long denied the indigenous communities of Guatemala. Among these human rights include the right to an identity, the right to life, the freedom to artistic creation and expression, the right to their primary language, and the right to participate in the social and political life of the nation. This series concludes with a banner briefly

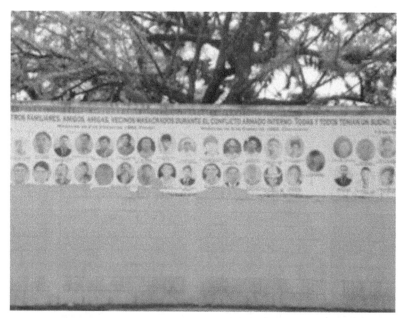

Figure 4.1. Names of Some of the Victims in the Outside Wall, Cementerio, Rabinal, 2017.
Source: Photo by the author

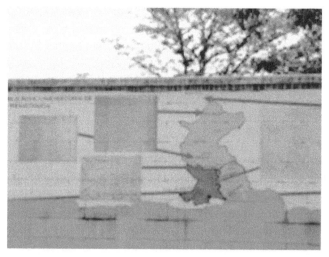

Figure 4.2. Map of Different Massacres in Baja Verapaz, Cementerio, Rabinal, 2017.
Source: Photo by the author

describing the events of the seven massacres under the headline "The History of the Beautiful Achí Rabinal Communities Were Without Violence" (translated, Rabinal, November 2019).

Within the cemetery and occupying an area in the rear of this burial ground are memorial monuments that document and commemorate the massacres that occurred. These individual memorials function as spaces for private reflection for survivors and the community as opposed to a more public and visibly educative purpose that the outside walls achieve. There are approximately seven memorial monuments where the victims of massacres from the Rabinal area are reburied. What do the memorial monuments tell us? Each memorial monument commemorates a specific massacre during the armed internal conflict and provides the date and the names of the victims reburied at the site. Many of the memorial monuments have a pictorial description that illustrates a scene depicting the violence of the massacre. Most of them also list those responsible for the violence citing the Guatemalan military and the civil patrols as perpetrators, even noting that those responsible enjoy their freedom while the community mourns. The memorial monuments also list the sponsors with ADIVIMA at the forefront of supporters. One memorial monument dedicated in May 1998 to the victims of the village of Panacal holds the remains of forty-seven campesinos who were tortured and murdered on September 20, 1981. One side of the memorial monument contains a worn, primitive-like drawing depicting both men and women hanging from trees while other victims are portrayed being thrown off the mountain—one victim is clearly a child. On the other side of the memorial is a plaque that inscribes the names of the martyrs with a notation indicating that they live on the community's memory and the community will not forget. The description on the plaque also calls for accountability of those the community holds responsible for the massacre, which they identify as the Guatemalan Army and the civil patrols from both Xococ and Vegas, Santo Domingo. The memorial's inscription recognizes the late Monsignor Gerardi as a defender of the country whose memory lives on. There are several additional memorials without pictorials that commemorate the victims from the communities of Chuategua, Pa Oj, and Chil Ixim from Rabinal, Baja Verapaz, who were massacred on November 24, 1982. Although they do not provide visual descriptions, they are consistent with the inscriptions on the other memorials in that they contain the inscribed names of the victims on the plaque identifying the massacres and the perpetrators who are consistently identified as the army and the civil patrols.

The memorial monument commemorating the multiple massacres of Río Negro is the most descriptive and most recognizable of the cemetery memorials. It is also the monument with the most active evidence of reflective and commemorative activity. On my multiple visits to the cemetery throughout the years, the Río Negro memorial consistently displayed various commemorative artifacts in the form of withering flower arrangements, mounds of candle wax, and the remains of food and other offerings. These offerings were in abundance in May 2018 and again in November 2019, shortly after the Día de los Muertos (Day of the Dead). The Río Negro massacres occurred during the height of the armed internal conflict that claimed the lives of nearly five hundred indigenous Maya Achí from communities along the Chixoy River basin in the Departments of Baja and Alta Verapaz.

As one of the largest and most recognizable of the Rabinal cemetery memorials, the Río Negro memorial commemorates two massacres associated with this community. One consistent representation on this memorial is the statement on the right side of the façade that indicts Colonel José Antonio Solares González and the civil patrols as the intellectual and physical actors responsible for the massacre of the women and children with the declaration that the survivors will never forget. The memorial has changed in appearance over the course of several visits to the area. One noticeable change from a visit in June 2018 to another in November 2019 was the addition of more visuals to the face of the memorial. This includes a historical narrative of the exhumations of the women and children from their clandestine graves in Pacoxom that began in late 1993. This inscription also notes the date, April 24, 1994, when the community reburied the victims; with the support of CONAVIGUA, they constructed a small monument in memory of the victims. The community attributes the military with destroying the original monument on June 2, 1994, and the narrative on the cemetery memorial visibly inscribes blame for the memorial's destruction on "*los asesinos.*" The narrative concludes by extolling the determination of the widows and orphan survivors who formed ADIVIMA, followed by a quote that reiterates the importance of historical memory for the community, "we will never forget the serious violations committed to us—the Maya Achís." Another change to the memorial's façade occurred in the illustration of the massacre of March 4, 1980, in which security agents working for INDE murdered seven members of the Río Negro community who were en route to the INDE offices (Johnston 2010, 350). The pictorial I photographed in 2017, now colorized from its former black and white sketch, features the seven massacre victims who stand beneath a written headline that recognized them as the first martyrs from Río Negro massacred for the construction of the Chixoy Dam (see figure 4.3).

While the visual representations on these private reflective memorials provide me, as outsider viewer, with images of the destruction of the communities in Rabinal, they do not depict the long-term cultural, emotional, and physical trauma suffered by the communities. Many surviving widows suffer from *tristeza*—a psychological condition not unlike post-traumatic stress disorder—and other physical and emotional distress such as physical

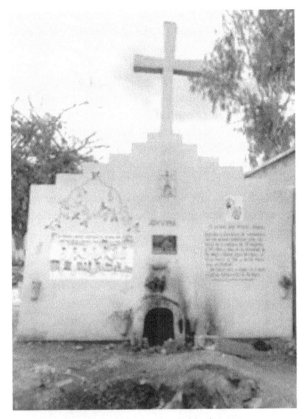

Figure 4.3. Río Negro Memorial, Cementerio, Rabinal, 2019.
Source: Photo by the author

pain, nightmares, unresolved grief, disturbing dreams, and fear (Vaughn and Cabrera 2009, xx; Garrard-Burnett 2015, xx). None of the cemetery memorials illustrate any expressions of the sexual violence that women experienced as part of the genocidal massacres. Nor do they reveal life post conflict and their struggles for transitional justice long after the peace accords were signed. Instead, the cemetery memorials are time-bound, and they capture the destruction of the communities during the scorched-earth campaign. They complete the rituals of death for those victims whose remains were identified and reinterred, and provide some measure of closure for survivors. As private reflective space, Bickford (2014, 504) reminds us that this form of a memory landscape does not have to offer a complete narrative because this space exists for survivors to commemorate and mourn their dead.

It remains a private space where survivors can return and connect with family members, a place where they can perform their religious rituals and commemorate loved ones in the hopes of gaining some measure of closure.

The same case has happened with many of the deaths from COVID-19; at the beginning many families were able to identify their bodies because of the restrictions they were buried in areas specifically assigned for COVID-19 victims. In the investigation about COVID-19, there where not murals or memorials identified particularly in Guatemala. One of the recent murals was completed in 2020 by EntreMundos, a "Guatemalan nonprofit organization, founded in 2001 to support organizations and groups that are committed to the fight against poverty and the defense and promotion of human rights for the country's most marginalized and vulnerable populations" (EntreMundos 2021). The non-governmental organization EntreMundos shared this photograph with me in July 2018; it is part of the mural for awareness created in Quetzaltenango in their facility in this area of Guatemala. It recognizes the work that members of the community and the lives of the deceased during the pandemic (see figure 4.4).

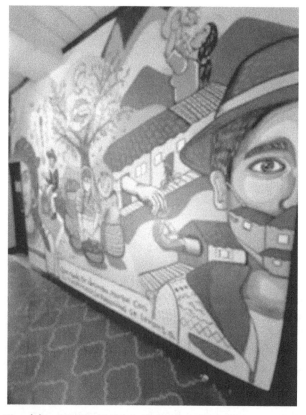

Figure 4.4. "Surviving COVID-19," EntredMundos, Quetzaltenango, Guatemala.
Source: La Asociación ENTREMUNDOS

EntreMundos specified that this mural was created to honor community resilience during the pandemic. They explained that the mural features a saleswoman:

> The saleswoman represents all those who sustained us during the pandemic; including the people who organised the cantonal [regional] markets. Thanks to their efforts, people who could not travel due to presidential decrees were able to feed themselves and their families, at the same time as supporting food producers, who were also affected by the pandemic. Also shown is a man speaking of planting vegetable gardens and medicinal herbs, both of which could be ways of combatting COVID-19 by strengthening immune defences and being healthy. (EntreMundos 2021)

This mural also brings attention to the use of medicinal herbs, taking into consideration that many of the Mayan communities relied on these herbal medicines and have learned their uses from their ancestors and are part of their culture. As a memorial to remember the victims of COVID-19, "This tribute seeks to remember those who lost their lives at work, and those who are still alive and making sacrifices; the image of the tree represents the hope that they will soon reunite with and be able to embrace their families, as many families are yet to be reunited" (EntreMundos 2021). This memorial educates and honors both the death and the living, and at the same time teach others of the sacrifices that were made having a private reflective space of remembrance.

CONCLUSION

Across the former conflict zones in Guatemala are dozens of private reflective memorials that serve as a place for survivors, relatives, and communities to mourn, heal, commemorate, and remember the victims of the violence that racked Guatemala during the height of the armed internal conflict; during the pandemic, there were specific COVID-19 burial areas. The creation of private reflective memorial continues in Guatemala today. Some function as private spaces where survivors can return and connect with family members, a place where they can perform their religious rituals and commemorate loved ones in the hopes of gaining some measure of closure. Many memorials dedicated to all those who perished will continue to be built as many remains have not been identified. Other families wait for COVID-19 pandemic victims to be returned to them and their communities for a proper burial. The pandemic continues and in the past months an increase of coronavirus cases has been recorded, leaving again the Mayan and poor communities vulnerable. Efforts of campaigns for vaccination and prevention have not reached all the Mayan indigenous communities.

REFERENCES

Association for the Integral Development of the Victims of Violence in the Verapaces (ADIVIMA). "History." n.d. derechos.net/adivima/en/history.htm

Bickford, Louis. "Memoryworks/Memory Works." In *Transitional Justice, Culture, and Society: Beyond Outreach*, edited by Clara Ramirez-Barat, 491–517. New York: Social Science Research Council, 2014.

Bol Chocooj, Cesar. "The State and its Responsibility to Indigenous People in the Face of the Coronavirus." June 24, 2020. https://www.culturalsurvival.org/news/ state-and-its-responsibility-indigenous-peoples-guatemala-face-coronavirus

Commission for Historical Clarification. *Guatemala Memory of Silence: Report of the Commission for Historical Clarification Conclusions and Recommendations.* February 25, 1999.

De Ros, Oliver. *Cementerio de La Verbena.* January 6, 2021. https://www.no-ficcion .com/project/olvidados-fallecidos-covid19

Doiron, Fabienne. "Indigenous Achí Widows' Experiences of Armed Conflict in Rabinal, Guatemala: Implications for Peace and Development in the Aftermath of La Violencia." Unpublished master's thesis, Saint Mary's University, 2007. https: //library2.smu.ca/bitstream/handle/01/22333/doiron_fabienne_masters_2007.PDF ?sequence=1&isAllowed=y

Doiron, Fabienne. "Widows, Mothers, Activists: Indigenous Achí Women's Experiences of La Violencia in Rabinal, Guatemala." *Journal of the Motherhood Initiative for Research and Community Involvement* 1, no. 1 (2010): 77–90. https: //jarm.journals.yorku.ca/index.php/jarm/article/view/30923/28352

Dupuis, Nieves Gómez. "Report of the Damage on the Health Mental derived of the Massacres of Plan de Sanchez for the Interamerican Court of Human Rights." Equipo de Estudios Comunitarios y Acción Psicosocial (ECAP), Guatemala: 2005, 1–15.

EntreMundos. "Painting in the Time of COVID-19: Art to Honour Community Resilience during the Pandemic." July 18, 2021. https://www.entremundos.org/ revista/culture/painting-in-the-time-of-covid-19/?lang=en

Garrard-Burnett, Virginia. "Living with Ghosts: Death, Exhumation, and Reburial Among the Maya in Guatemala." *Latin American Perspectives* 42, no.3 (2015): 180–92.

Gobierno de Guatemala. "Tablero COVID-19 Guatemala: Situación del COVID-19 en Guatemala." May 19, 2023. https://tableros.mspas.gob.gt/covid/

Gobierno de Guatemala. "Tablero de Alertas Covid-19." May 19, 2023. https:// covid19.gob.gt/datos/semaforo/14Abril23/Historico_Alertas_mapas_del_31_de_ marzo_al_13_de_abril_del_2023_A.pdf

Green, Linda. "Fear as a Way of Life." *Cultural Anthropology* 9, no. 2 (1994): 227–56.

Henderson, Erica, Catherine Nolin, and Fredy Peccerelli. "Dignifying a Bare Life and Making Place through Exhumation: Cobán CREOMPAZ Former Military Garrison, Guatemala." *Journal of Latin American Geography* 13, no. 2 (2014): 97–116.

Instituto Nacional de Estadística. "Población maya por comunidad lingüística." Resultados del Censo 2018. El Instituto Nacional de Estadística (INE). https://www .censopoblacion.gt/explorador

Johnston, Barbara Rose. "Chixoy Dam Legacies: The Struggle to Secure Reparation and the Right to Remedy in Guatemala." *Water Alternatives* 3, no. 2 (2010): 341–61.

Menchú, Sofía. "Nadie puede llorar a las víctimas de la pandemia." *No-Ficción.* January 6, 2021. https://www.no-ficcion.com/project/olvidados-fallecidos-covid19

Moffett, Luke. "Collective Reparations and Plan de Sanchez." VIMEO video, 5:14. August 20, 2018. https://reparations.qub.ac.uk/plan-de-sanchez-massacre-video/

Museo Comunitario Rabinal Achí (MCRA). *Oj K'aslik, Estamos Vivos: Recuperación de la Memoria Histórica de Rabinal (1944–1996).* Rabinal: MCRA, 2003.

Peace Brigades International (PBI) Guatemala. "The Impact of COVID-19 in Communities Accompanied by PBI." December 2021. https://pbi-guatemala.org/en /news/2022-02/impact-covid-19-communities-accompanied-pbi#sdfootnote2sym

Proyecto Interdiocesano Recuperación de la Memoria Histórica (Guatemala), Catholic Institute for International Relations, and Latin America Bureau. Guatemala, Never Again! / REMHI, Recovery of Historical Memory Project; the official report of the Human Rights Office, Archdiocese of Guatemala. New York: Orbis Books, 1999.Tomuschat, Christian. Foreward: *In Memory of Silence: The Guatemalan Truth Commission Report*, edited by Daniel Rothenburg, xv-xli. New York: Palgrave Macmillan, 2012. Print.

Rothenberg, Daniel, ed. *Memory of Silence: The Guatemalan Truth Commission Report.* New York: Palgrave Macmillan, 2012.

Sanford, Victoria. *Buried Secrets: Truth and Human Rights in Guatemala.* London: Palgrave Macmillan, 2003.

Stewart, Julie. "When Local Troubles Become Transnational: The Transformation of a Guatemalan Indigenous Rights Movement." *Mobilization: An International Journal* 9, no. 3 (2004): 259–78.

Stewart, Julie. "A Measure of Justice: The Rabinal Human Rights Movement in Post-War Guatemala." *Qualitative Sociology* 31 (2008): 231–50.

Vaughn, Lisa M., and Gabriela de Cabrera. "Left Alone, the Widows of the War: Trauma Reframed through Community Empowerment in Guatemala." In *Feminist Conversations: Women, Trauma, and Empowerment in Post-Transitional Societies*, edited by Dovile Byudryte, Lisa M. Vaughn, and Natalya T. Reigg, 91–99. Lanham: University Press of America, 2009.

Webb, Meghan, and Miguel Cuj. "Guatemala's Public Health Messaging in Mayan Languages during the COVID-19 pandemic. *Journal of Indigenous Social Development* 9, no. 3 (2020): 102–09. https://journalhosting.ucalgary.ca/index.php /jisd/article/view/70808/54418

World Health Organization. "Guatemala: WHO Coronavirus Disease (Covid-19) Dashboard with Vaccination Data." n.d. Accessed July 15, 2022. https://covid19 .who.int/region/amro/country/gt.

Zur, Judith N. *Violent Memories: Mayan War Widows in Guatemala.* Boulder: Westview Press, 1998.

Chapter Five

Between Life and Death

Practices of Healing of the Ecuadorian Siona Nationality as a Political Spirituality

María Fernanda Solórzano Granada

Capitalist rationality must be understood as a civilizational model of domination, violence, dispossession, coloniality, and hegemony. It is a way of life based on mercantile rationality, so the denial and destruction of the spiritual dimension of the native people leads to the breaking of the interrelationships with nature and the environment.

The interrelation between the indigenous population and nature/environment is a form of healing and spirituality[1] that has a political dimension because it has allowed the subjugated original people to survive. This relationship with nature/environment as a form of healing is transmitted through the wisdom of grandmothers and grandfathers in the ancestral memory, myths, and the ceremony of sacred plants.

This interrelation between indigenous and nature/environment evidences their feelings, thoughts, and practices into their cosmos that allows them to constitute themselves as a collective political subjectivity; that is, as political subjects in the face of extractivist processes. For this reason, their sacred plants ceremony and their medicinal plants have more than a simple vision of the world; it is a way to re-existence and resistance (Walsh 2013).

The Siona Indigenous Nationality has its territories in Ecuador and Colombia. In Ecuador, their communities are in Shushufindi, Cuyabeno, and Putumayo, in the Sucumbíos province. Its territory is made up of two geographically separated areas and with different legal situations—the ancestral territory and the shared territory—with a total extension of approximately

164,552.95 hectares.[2] In Ecuador, there are eight Siona communities: four communities settled on the banks of the Aguarico River (*Orahuëaya*, *Aboquëhuira*, *Biaña*, and *Soto Tsiaya*) and four communities located on the Cuyabeno River (San Victoriano, *Tarabëaya*, *Sëoquëaya*, and Puerto Bolívar). According to the last community census, there is a population of 682 Siona people (Organización de la Nacionalidad Indígena Siona del Ecuador ONISE 2021).

The Siona territory is a complexity of differentiated interrelations between humans, non-humans, spirits, the state, evangelical religion, and the extractive industry (Solórzano 2020a). The current configuration of the Siona communities is the result of processes of colonization and coloniality (Quijano 2000) since the arrival of the Summer Institute of Linguistics (SIL) in the 1950s,[3] the State Colonization Law in the 1970s, and extractives projects.[4] In this context, the Siona people live in completeness and complementarity, which is not only an attempt to (re)assemble the social to nature as proposed by the French rationality of Latour (2008), but rather, through their traditional practices. They have different cultural practices of healing that become processes of insurgency.

When I met the wise grandfather[5] Carlos,[6] he was seventy-seven years old; he was born and lived in *Orehuëya* community, located on the banks of the Aguarico River, on the northern border of Ecuador and Colombia. During my first year of fieldwork, I heard many stories about him: "Grandpa Carlos is the most powerful shaman in Aguarico," "Grandfather is the only one who still knows how to communicate with all the spirits of our territory," "Carlos is the one who knows how to heal from all diseases," and "Carlos has the wisdom of *yagé* (ayahuasca)." I experienced his wisdom during the *yagé* ceremony, where I could feel in my body the biocosmic alterity (Guerrero 2018) between humans and non-humans.

When I met Grandpa Samuel, he was seventy-nine years old; he was born in the Aguarico River. He and his family built the community called *Soto Tsiaya*. His story captivated me because Samuel's life represents an assemblage (Deleuze and Guattari 2004; Verschoor and Torres 2016) between evangelical religion and Siona spirituality.[7]

When SIL arrived in Siona territories, Samuel was one of the first indoctrinated to evangelical catechism. In the 1970s, he was a teacher at the first Siona School. From then on, he maintained his practice of evangelization with the children of his community, but despite professing an evangelical religion, he used to use a wide variety of *ujas* (healing and protection songs) and sacred plants for healing.

The influence of the North American evangelical missionaries caused internal conflicts in the communities and spiritual conflicts in some people;

for example, Grandfather Samuel chose not to continue with the *yagé* ceremony, but to practice healing *ujas*.

In 2020, the World Health Organization declared COVID-19 a pandemic. In May, I heard the first news about the deaths of Amazonian indigenous people due to SARS-COV-2. In that context, the Siona people decided to "close their communities" and turn to their natural medicine.

> We do not want anyone to come to our communities. In our communities, we are avoiding panic, we do not want that the doctors tell us that we are sick and take us to the hospital, because when we are in the hospital they do not give us food or treatment. The doctors only give oxygen and serums, and we have no options to use our medicinal plants. That is why, we decided to use our own treatments and medicine. That is the only thing that will heal and take care of us. (chat with Javier, young Siona, May 2020)

In June 2020, Grandfather Samuel passed away. His death could be associated to the pandemic, but according to his relatives, it was due to some "sorcery." In November 2020, Grandfather Carlos also passed away. When I asked his grandson if he died due to COVID-19, the answer was: "wise grandparents do not die from Western diseases, grandparents die for struggle between good spirits and bad spirits." This is the main conflict since the historical background of oppression persists in indigenous imaginaries, thus the decision to bring back to the traditional ways is a cultural and symbolically political.

Langdon (1996) points out there is no specific name to express the force that enables the Siona people to heal when stalked by a spirit that causes disease. That vital force could be the heart (*dekoyo*) because it is the center of life in the physical body, and when a Siona is dying, it is the last part that remains warm. In some narratives, when a Siona dies, his heart takes the shape of a bird. Nevertheless, when a wise grandfather dies, his heart flies like a great macaw. The vital force of the heart abides and accompanies the Siona people in interrelation with other non-human beings. The Siona force does not die but interconnects with other beings or spirits. As Grandfather Carlos said: "I am like a cicada that rejuvenates and leaves his spirit in the jungle" (personal conversation, August 2019).

In this context, I wonder how the Siona nationality lives and feels the diseases. For Siona people, life and death are interrelated with their healing and protection practices through their healing songs (*ujas*) and sacred plants, which are actions "to protect the world from the evil spirits that exist in the jungle and to take care of the Siona Nationality" (personal conversation with wise Grandfather Samuel, February 2018).

THE *UJAS* AS HEALING SONGS

There is an interrelationship between all living beings in the Siona territory, which expresses their spirituality. This spirituality materializes, mainly, in the *yagé* ceremony and the *ujas* prayer. Also, the wise grandparents are protectors and caretakers of the territory and life through their connection with all the spirits of the *airo* (jungle).

The Siona translate *ujas* like a prayer, not songs as they appear in some of the ethnographies on Amazonian indigenous peoples.[8] This translation comes from the evangelization process from SIL. These prayers are repetitions in a low voice, like mantras, and they are the way of communication between humans and non-humans, as Grandpa Samuel said, "*uja* are transmitted by the spirits that is why it has a language that sometimes it is not understood" (personal conversation with Grandfather Samuel, April 2018). In other words, these prayers become channels of cosmic information through which wise grandparents walk to meet the spirits. In the Aguarico communities, if a person knows more *ujas*, they are more respected because it means they know the wisdom to heal.

The *ujas* are varied. The Siona people use them for the care of pregnancies, to control menstruation, for home births, fertility, to cause abortions, to have good hunting and fishing, to heal body aches, to fall in love, to treat respiratory diseases, avoid "sorcery," and to have fortune. When *ujas* are pronounced, the Siona people speak with the spirits of plants, crops, and animals. Descola (2005) explained that the songs of the Achuar indigenous people are like melodies that transcend all linguistic barriers and turn each animal or plant into a subject that produces meanings. The *ujas* should be repeated as a prayer or song, because their sounds and words allow to make a connection with the spirits.

The wisdom of the *ujas* is the greatest treasure for the Siona people, for this reason they are very cautious of sharing this knowledge.

> It is difficult for us to learn *ujas*. When we drink *yocó* and *yagé* [sacred plants] we learn *uja* little by little because it is a different language, it is an ancient *baicoca* [Siona language]. "B*aaina*" [Siona's god] created the *uja*. It is like learning another language, I do not know what some words mean, and we have to memorize it. I have written down in a notebook some *ujas* that my grandfather told me, and I want to learn because they help for everything. Although it is difficult, my dad told me that it is important to learn them.
>
> There are many *ujas* for example, "*Ñamami uja*" that is used if a stingray fish hurts us, it calms the pain and the bleeding stops. *Baaina* [Siona's god] is invoked, he is the creator of all prayers and the *ujas* calm the pain.

We pray the "*Wa'ti tëto uja*" when there is an accident. My cousin broke his head and this *uja* does work. (personal conversation with Javier, young Siona, March 2018)

There is also the "*Siba Uja*"; it is the *uja* before giving birth, when a woman is eight months pregnant, we give her natural medicines, washes her uterus, and we sing this *uja to* not suffer at the time of give birth. (personal conversation with Grandmother Adela, March 2018)

In the *Soto Tsiaya* community, even though Grandfather Samuel was an evangelical, he firmly believed in the healing power of the *uja*. These expressions continue to have force despite of the rationalization of the evangelical religion that prohibits these practices. As Grandfather Samuel said, "the *ujas* are secrets, it is our ancestral language, and it cannot be translated, it is learned because it is repeated. The *ujas* are to heal or to harm, that is why we have to be careful" (personal conversation with Grandfather Samuel, August 2018).

Each spirit in nature has its own *uja* that the wise grandparents and grandmothers must master. These prayers are learned through the spirit of the sacred plants, in dreams, in ceremonies, or from one wise grandfather to another person. Generally, this *cosmocimiento*[9] (Guerrero 2018) is transmitted from man to man, but some women know a few *ujas* because they are useful for childbirth and healing diseases. Unfortunately, the generation between thirty and fifty years old knows a limited repertoire of *ujas*, while the younger population is just learning some.

Both the *ujas* and the sacred plants (*yagé* and *yocó*) are the channels between the spirits of the *airo* (jungle) and the wise grandparents. The *ujas* and the sacred plants have a relationship that allows the Siona people to continue with their *biocosmic alterity*, as expressed in the following story.

Baaina [primal being, Sionas'god] lived in our territory and drunk *yagé* and *yocó*. Formerly, the tapir was a person, one day she pricked her leg and *baaina* tried to help her and asked her to kick. In that moment *baaina* turned a person into a tapir. *Baaina* turned all the people who lived in our territory into animals. Animals were created from people, for this reason *yagé* drinkers transform into tapirs, *guanganas*, and tigers. Only when we drink *yagé* we can transform into an animal, because *baaina* left his spirit in *yagé*.

Animals do not become human; they could never become human because they were already human. On the other hand, we transform into animals because animals have a spirit (*mai joyo*) [soul that is transmitted] that is why when we drink *yagé* we speak as an animal. (personal conversation with Aquíles, Siona leader, August 2018)

This myth testifies that all the animals were people who were transformed to have the peculiar appearance of animals that they are now. There is an original condition of human beings in all inhabits the cosmos; in certain conflicts, they transform themselves into animals, into new bodies. Thus, everything (human and non-human) are originally similar beings who, due to some conflict, become different.

Cayón (2010) proposes the category "cosmoproduction" to understand the bond of life between all beings, "as an intellectual and practical manifestation of a unique and complex epistemology, a politics of the cosmos, and an ethics of a people" (Cayón 2010, 265). In addition, Cayón (2010) mentions that the relationships between humans and non-humans in the cosmos of the Amazonian indigenous people have a social and spiritual character. That is, all plants and animals are considered as people with human qualities, which can change to transform themselves into various beings. The social relations "are regulated by a principle of symmetric reciprocity, for example, if you hunt in places that are the *malocas* (houses) of the animals without making a shamanic negotiation or healing, it is the same that entering a *maloca* of another person and kill an individual or steal a woman" (Cayón 2010, 202).

Related to the cosmoproduction category, there is the concept of "cosmopolitics" proposed by Stengers (2007). This category talks about multiversal interaction[10] with human and non-human alterities (Aparicio 2015). The concepts of cosmopolitics and cosmoproduction[11] propose that these interrelations go beyond the socio-political sphere, expanding the sociality of human beings to a space of interaction with non-human groups. In other words, these concepts propose that in the life of the Amazonian people there are multiple connections and articulations. In this sense, the cosmos-territory has a spiritual dimension, where identity allows one to meet otherness that is not only reduced to the human, but to all beings in the world, that is a biocosmic alterity (Guerrero 2018).

Langdon (1996) affirms that for the Siona people, spirits or *wati* are neutral, although some are potentially aggressive or can cause harm. The *wati* live in the jungle, in rivers, in the sky, in animals, etc.

> For the Siona, reality has two "sides," and many entities transform into others depending on which side they are on. This side of reality, *in kãko*, is the side we normally see, and plants, animals, people have a shape. On the other side, which is usually reached through ingestion of hallucinogens or through dreams, they can appear as other beings. In dreams and visions, human beings often take the form of birds. Animals, particularly the jaguar, anaconda, and peccaries, appear as humans. The fish in the river appear like corn. The Sun is seen as a star on this side, but is a person on the other. The idea of transformation is

central to the Siona worldview. The other side is a transformation of this side. (Langdon 1996, 64)

Wise grandparents are those who are on both sides of Siona reality and visit the different universes and worlds of spirits. They have healing and transformative powers, and they are mediators between the two sides. As leaders they must influence the "other side" to act in favor or well-being of their group/ communities.

The power of the wise grandparents is expressed in a physical substance called *dau*, which grows within their body, allowing them to differentiate themselves from other human beings. However, the *dau* also expresses a certain kind of delicacy that must be cared of. "The *dau* is the source of the shaman's power, but it also makes his body delicate and susceptible to damage through contamination" (Langdon 1996, 64). This vital force must be nourished with several ceremonies of *yagé*, with *ujas* and medicinal plants, and also to the restrictions of not consuming salt and sexual abstinence. While it is true that the *dau* is powerful, it is also fragile to the "curses" of other grandparents, menstruation, or diseases caused by bad spirits.

Therefore, when a wise grandfather dies, like Samuel and Carlos, their spirits linger for some time. Occasionally, they choose not to "die" and permanently transform into an animal. Although the deaths of the wise grandparents during the pandemic could be associated with COVID-19, for the Siona people these deaths represent spiritual struggles and transcendence.

SACRED PLANTS AS A VITAL MEDICINE

Since the middle of the twentieth century, anthropology has carried out countless studies on shamanic knowledge, its practices, and sacred plants (Langdon 2013). Different ethnographies recognize that plants have wisdom and power, which is inseparable from healing, protection, and spirituality.

Specifically, the *yagé* has spiritual and healing power in the life of the Siona people. This plant is considered as the great healer of diseases. During my fieldwork, I was able to collect several testimonies about its healing power. In the Puerto Bolívar community, one of the wise grandfathers testified to his wife's healing with sacred plants. "My wife was in the hospital in Quito for almost three weeks, she had leukemia, and the doctor told me there was no cure. I took her out of the hospital and brought her to the community. With seven *yagé* ceremonies she was cured" (personal conversation with Grandpa Israel, August 2018).

According to the version of Israel's wife, Marcia, she overcame leukemia thanks to the *yagé* treatment.

The pus was coming out of my body, I suffered for five months, and the doctor told me I was going to die. My husband took me to the Marco Vinicio Iza Hospital in Quito; Israel arrived at the Hospital and took me out of there to treat me with *yagé*. He did seven *yagé* ceremonies and the leukemia disappeared. The doctors made medical exams, and I had already cured. I spent almost 800 dollars on western medicine that did not cure me, but I spent nothing with *yage*. (personal conversation with Marcia, August 2018)

However, *yagé* is not the only sacred healing plant; *yocó* (paullinia yoco) is another important liana in the life of the Siona nationality. This sacred plant is consumed in the early morning. A wise grandfather scrapes it off and drinks the juice with water; he is in charge of its preparation and distribution to the family.

When the Siona people drink *yocó*, it is the time to talk about their daily routines, past life, or schedule future events, but, above all, it is time to teach and learn the *ujas* (healing prayers). It is also a precious moment for the Siona people because this sacred plant transmits energy to work all day. Unfortunately, *yocó* consumption has drastically decreased in recent years; for example, in *Soto Tsiaya* community, it is not common to find in their crops.

Yocó is used to have energy, not to be hungry, and to regain our spirit. It helps to have energy to hunt. It is good for diabetes and for many diseases. When we drink *yocó*, we talk about our hunting stories, but also gives us the strength to work, to weave and to make our hammocks. (personal conversation with Grandfather Delio del Cuyabeno, August 2018)

I had the opportunity to drink *yocó* on several occasions in Cuyabeno and Aguarico communities. I experienced the healing power of this plant. I had spent two days with severe stomachache caused by gastritis. Israel proposed to cure me with several *yocó* drinks, which were effective in the treatment for gastritis.

Fernanda, I am going to cure you, but you must drink *yocó* for 14 days to heal. The *yocó* is good because it removes all diseases. The doctor cannot cure evil spirits that cause harm, but when we drink *yocó* the evil spirit do not live in our body. In our language, we say *maju* [bad spirit]; we must drink *yocó* so that *maju* does not reach us. (personal conversation with Grandpa Israel, August 2018)

These narratives evidence their healing spirituality that persists in Siona cosmoexistence.[12] Western medicine does not understand how to "cure evil spirits," while the Siona people know how to dialogue with the *maju* and how to protect themselves. The sacred plants have the healing spirits; they teach the wise grandmothers and grandfathers about healing and protection. Therefore, in a world where spirituality is still condemned, symbolic and political insurgency practices survive to perpetuate life.

The Siona nationality knows that invisible entities inhabit their vast territory. They know it when the sing *ujas* and drink sacred plants. All spirits are behind the visible world and are the cause of diseases. The Siona's conception of disease is similar to the various Pan-Amazonian people. For them, diseases have symptoms outside the human body, which indicate the causes of the disease. The cause of diseases is "sorcery" or an evil spirit (*maju*).

They understand the death of the grandparents Samuel and Carlos as a relationship with these "bad" spirits. The diseases associated with witchcraft are motivated by the wise grandparents from a certain spirit or *wati* when there are social conflicts, anger, or when someone breaks a taboo. These spirits attack a person when they have little physical resistance. In that sense, the same wise grandparents are in charge of communicating and reaching agreements with the spirits to improve the health of the person.

Siona people believe that the COVID-19 disease is associated with external factors produced by the "Western world," thus the negotiation with the spirits is much more powerful. The wise grandparents should use various strategies and different medicinal plants to face the pandemic.

According to the communal census, the main causes of death in the Aguarico zone is "sorcery or evil spirits," while in the Cuyabeno communities, the causes of death are related to "Western diseases" such as pneumonia and cancer (Organización de la Nacionalidad Indígena Siona del Ecuador ONISE 2021). This difference is due to the Cuyabeno communities having a much stronger evangelization process than in Aguarico. Evangelism has condemned spirituality and traditional forms of healing.

THE RETURN OF SPIRITUALITY DURING THE COVID-19 PANDEMIC

During my fieldwork with the Siona nationality from 2016 to 2020, I evidenced a high percentage of the population, especially the young, who do not practice ceremonies and *ujas*, and do not know the use of sacred plants. The greatest concern of the older adult population is the non-transmission of their traditions and wisdom. The death of the wise grandparents Samuel and Carlos turned out to be events of great importance in the sense of knowing who will transmit and continue with their practices and knowledge.

It was precisely during the pandemic that the Siona's ways of healing were revitalized, as well as the application of their traditional practices and self-organization in their territory.

During this pandemic, we have stuck together as a family. The families that were abroad came to the territory, we always stood firm with our natural medicine, mainly with *yagé*, which is very important to us. In my case, I suffered the symptoms of COVID, I was very sick, I drank *yagé*, and the symptoms were relieved. I completed my treatment by using other plants and I began to recover, and I did the same with my parents. In the community, we only use native plants. We use that type of medicine that helped us to control COVID. (telephone conversation with indigenous leader, Aquíles, June 2021)

On the other hand, the absence of the Ecuadorian government was evidenced in priority issues such as health in the Amazonian indigenous communities during the pandemic. Indigenous territories are not a priority in emergency issues, but they are very important for extractive purposes, specifically the northern Amazon of Ecuador because it is the largest place of oil production.

In my community, there was a total absence of the State, when there were many sick people, we requested the government to help us, but our communities are far away and it was difficult to deliver supplies. We decided taking care of each other.

We know that the government uses the pandemic to isolate us, but at the same time, they take the opportunity to make concessions to oil companies. For this reason, we have said that we should not be afraid of COVID, but we do have to respect it. We say that when it rains hard and we are in the jungle, we cannot wait for that rain to calm down; we look for a safe place. The COVID has been like that constant rain. We could not wait with our arms crossed, waiting for the government to help us until the pandemic finishes. We continue to search for strategies to take care of ourselves, without fear but with respect because not all of us are in the same capacity to face the COVID. (telephone conversation with an indigenous leader, Aquíles, June 2021)

The main strategy to face the pandemic in the Siona communities is the inclusion of traditional medicine as a form of healing. Thus, the revitalization of their traditional knowledge became one of their main strengths to face COVID-19.

We realized that Western medicine is useless and we decided to live with our own medicine to face the COVID. There are several testimonies of people that are alive because they did not go to the hospital but, rather, they used our traditional medicine. For example, the case of the Siona grandmother from Putumayo who was very sick in the hospital, we took her out of the hospital and applied traditional medicine to save our grandmother.

We say that the COVID is not a problem for us. This illness made us understand that we have been losing our sense of community and our traditions. Now we save ourselves with our own ways of healing. COVID taught us that our traditions are very valuable for our survival. (telephone conversation with indigenous leader, Aquíles, June 2021)

The pandemic allowed the revitalization of the ancestral practices, values, and wisdom regarding care and protection to perpetuate their lives. Likewise, the death of the two wise grandparents implied an agitation and reminder about the need to revitalizing their wisdoms.

CONCLUSIONS: THE SYMBOLIC INSURGENCY AND POLITICAL SPIRITUALITY

Siona people believe that disease/health, life/death, and human/non-human are interrelated as interdependencies within their territory where their sacred healing plants, *ujas*, and ceremonies are conductors of protection and healing. Their spirituality is in their economic, cultural, religious, family, and health practices; therefore, it is a political issue because it allows its survival under colonial structures, such as evangelization. Therefore, these healing and protection practices are forms of symbolic insurgency and a political spirituality for re-existence in the face of colonial contexts (Walsh 2013).

During the pandemic, the healing and protection practices from the Siona people were revitalized to give continuity to their "practices that are determined to continue celebrating their existence, despite the looting of their material and symbolic resources" (Solórzano 2020b, 81). In this sense, the pandemic allowed them to become political subjects in the face of colonialist processes (Quijano 2000).

Indigenous medicine considers the human being as an undivided unit between spirit-body-mind-territory; therefore, for the Siona people death/life meant a return to interrelation with non-human spirits to generate communal well-being during the pandemic. Thus, their spirituality becomes an insurgency not only symbolic but also political, because the political has subjectivities that lead to territorial protection and a defense of life (Guerrero 2019).

The *yagé* ceremony, the *ujas*, and the sacred plants are an expression of the spiritualties and wisdoms for the Siona people who live ceremonially, symbolically, festively, and affectively in an interrelation with the cosmos (Guerrero 2018). The *ujas* and the sacred plants are a vital memory.

I affirm that the Siona practices of healing allow the perpetuation of their spirituality, their system of protection, and their sense of life or destruction. This text evidences how the Siona spirituality face the coronavirus pandemic, diseases, and sense of life/death. Their wise grandparents and their healing practices are a manifestation of biocosmic alterity, that is, the interdependence that dialogues with all beings.

CONVERSATIONS[13]

Javier Biaguaje
Samuel Piaguaje
Carlos Yiyocuro
Adela Suale
Aquíles Biaguaje
Israel Yiyocuro
Marcia Piyaguaje
Delio Yiyocuro

NOTES

1. In this spiritual dimension, all beings are interrelated. As Pitarch (1996) mentioned in his book *Ch'ulel. An Ethnography of Tzeltal Souls*, the person is composed of several beings, unlike the modern conception in which someone must have a single identity.

2. 164,552.95 hectares represents 406,619.19 acres.

3. The SIL arrived in the Siona territory in 1951 for a Christian indoctrination. SIL was founded by William Cameron Townsend in 1930, after World War II. This institute established the Radio Service and the project called "Jungle Aviation" to enter into isolated indigenous populations. SIL presented itself as an organization for the study of the languages of indigenous people; its work was not exclusively to study indigenous languages to translate the Bible, but to convert indigenous to be leaders of the church and carry forward the evangelical mission. But evangelization goes far beyond the theological indoctrination. SIL brought the values of capitalism, including individual wage labor, as well as discourses from a fervent anti-communist and pro-American attitude that was a necessary component of the process of becoming a Christian. SIL missionaries initiated the colonization of knowledge in the Amazon region. The missionaries translated the Bible into the Siona language (*baicoca*), built indoctrination schools, and joined clans to formed communities. In the process of conversion to Christianity, the missionaries condemned the spiritual world of the Siona people and established the Western family as the nuclear base for social production. SIL was expelled from Ecuador in 1981 by President Jaime Roldós, but its work continued in various parts of the Amazon and Siona territory.

4. In 1970, the Ecuadorian Institute for Agrarian Reform and Colonization decreed the Colonization Law to declare the Amazon as "waste lands," which generated the appropriation of 42 percent of indigenous ancestral territories by oil companies and population from other cities (Eberhart 1998). In addition, this law allowed the exploitation of oil, wood, and palm oil.

5. Quoting the words of Grandfather Carlos: "Shaman is not in our language; the foreign people called us shaman. Foreigners call us shaman, but shaman in our *Baicoca* language is *yagé cuquë* (who drinks *yagé*) or wise grandfather." In this, text

I will use "wise grandfather" to refer to the grandparents who practice the *yagé* ceremony (ayahuasca).

6. The author of this paper changed the names of the interviewees due to ethics policies.

7. French philosophers Gilles Deleuze and Félix Guattari in their text "A Thousand Plateaus wrote the concept of assemblage. Capitalism and Schizophrenia" (2004 [1980]). Also, this analytic category was written by the philosopher Manuel De Landa in two important books *A New Philosophy of Society* (2006) and *Assemblage Theory* (2016). The idea of assemblage is a way of ordering heterogeneous categories that work together in a certain time/space. For Deluze and Guattari, there are no predetermined hierarchies. Furthermore, all entities (humans, animals, things, and matters) have the same ontological status to initiate an assemblage. I consider that the category of assemblage is useful from its most descriptive sense based on Deluze and Guattari's theory, that is, from the meaning of a contingent set of practices, objects, people, and non-humans, that can be differentiated and cannot be similar, but can be combined to create new spaces or practices. I explain how ontological incompatible elements confront and incorporate with a capitalist reality legitimized by Western rationality. The assemblage proposal analyzes the multiplicity of practices and realities where the actors must face dilemmas of use of common resources or their integration to access to capitalism and religion.

8. Aparicio (2015) and Descola (2005) translate these expressions like songs.

9. Knowledge of the cosmos.

10. A similar category is "multinaturalist" proposed by Viveiros de Castro (2002).

11. As Müller (2015) mentions, the relationship between humans and non-humans has been called "ontological politics" by Mol (1999), "dingpolitik" by Latour (2008), or "cosmopolitics" by Stengers (2005). These concepts have some differences between them, especially to analyze a simile of the socio-political life of indigenous populations that are reproduced in the spiritual field. In this chapter, I use these concepts from their most descriptive notion, which is, the interrelationships, interdependencies, and connections between humans and non-humans that guide their practices, identities, and that, in a certain way, are reproduced on the human and spiritual level.

12. "The concept of cosmoexistence criticizes the category of cosmovision that prioritizes the cognitive way of knowing reality. For indigenous people, their wisdom about the cosmos is not only cognitively or rationally, but affectively, experientially, ceremonially, spiritually through all their senses and corporeality, and not only from vision" (Guerrero 2018, 23).

13. The author of this chapter changed the names of the interviewees due to ethics policies.

REFERENCES

Aparicio, Miguel. *Presas del veneno. Cosmopolítica y transformaciones Suruwaha (Amazonía occidental)*. Quito: Abya Yala, 2015.

Cayón, Luis. "Penso, logo crio. A teoria makuna do mundo." Doctoral thesis, Universidad de Brasilia, 2010.

Deleuze, Gilles, and Félix Guattari. *Mil Mesetas. Capitalismo y esquizofrenia.* Valencia: Pre-Textos, 2004.

DeLanda, Manuel. *A New Philosophy of Society: Assemblage Theory and Social Complexity.* London: Continuum, 2006.

DeLanda, Manuel. *Assemblage Theory.* London: Edinburgh University Press, 2016.

Descola, Philippe. *Las lanzas del crepúsculo. Relatos jíbaros. Alta Amazonía.* Buenos Aires: Fondo de Cultura Económico de Argentina, 2005.

Eberhart, Nicolás. *Transformaciones Agrarias en el Frente de Colonización de la Amazonía Ecuatoriana.* Quito: Abya Yala, 1998.

Guerrero, Patricio. *La chakana del corazonar. Desde las espiritualidades y las sabidurías insurgentes de Abya Yala.* Quito: Abya Yala, 2018.

Guerrero, Patricio. "Después de mi tiempo otro tiempo vendrá y ustedes cogerán leña de otro tiempo. Corazonando las insurgencias runas, los procesos políticos, la universidad y la interculturalidad." In *Interculturalidad. Problemáticas y perspectivas diversas*, edited by Fernando Garcés and Rubén Bravo, 123–66. Quito: Abya Yala, 2019.

Langdon, Esther. "¿Mueren en realidad los chamanes?: narraciones de los siona sobre chamanes muertos." *Alteridades* 6 (1996): 61–75.

Langdon, Esther. "La eficacia simbólica de los rituales: del ritual a la 'performance.'" In *Ayahuasca y Salud*, edited by Beatriz Labate and Carlos Bouso, 88–119. Barcelona: La Liebre de Marzo, 2013.

Latour, Bruno. *Reensamblar lo social. Una introducción a la teoría del actor-red.* Buenos Aires: Manantial, 2008.

Mol, Annemarie. "Ontological Politics. A Word and Some Questions". *The Sociological Review* 47 (1999): 74–89.

Müller, Martin. "Assemblages and Actor-networks: Rethinking Socio-material Power, Politics and Space," *Geography Compass* (2015): 27–41.

Organización de la Nacionalidad Indígena Siona del Ecuador ONISE. *Plan de Vida de la Nacionalidad Indígena Siona del Ecuador.* Tena: Empresa Pública IKIAM-EP, 2021.

Pitarch, Pedro. *Ch'ulel. Una etnografía de las almas tzeltales.* México: Fondo de Cultura Económica, 1996.

Quijano, Aníbal. "Colonialidad del poder, eurocentrismo y América Latina." In *La colonialidad del saber: eurocentrismo y ciencias sociales. Perspectivas Latinoamericanas*, edited by Edgardo Lander, 201–46. Buenos Aires: CLACSO, Consejo Latinoamericano de Ciencias Sociales, 2000.

Solórzano Granada, María Fernanda. "Espiritualidad en el airo (selva): un territorio insurgente en la nacionalidad siona del Ecuador." *Rile/Jile—An International Peer* 6 (2020a): 75–97.

Solórzano Granada, María Fernanda. "Los sionas de Soto Tsiaya y su territorio (*sia'ye ba'iji mai airo*): ensamblajes e interfaces sociales en su cosmoexistencia." Doctoral thesis, Centro de Investigaciones y Estudios Superiores en Antropología Social, 2020b.

Stengers, Isabelle. "The Cosmopolitical Proposal." In *Making Things Public: Atmospheres of Democracy*, edited by Bruno Latour and Peter Weibel, 994–1003. Cambridge: MIT Press, 2005.

Stengers, Isabelle. "La Proposition Cosmopolitique." In *L'Emergence des Cosmopolitiques*, edited by Jaacques Lolive and Olivier Soubeyran, 45–68. Paris: La Découverte, 2007.

Verschoor, Gerard, and Camillo Torres. "Mundos equivocados: cuando la 'abundancia' y la 'carencia' se encuentran en la Amazonía colombiana." *Íconos* 54 (2016): 71–86.

Viveiros de Castro, Eduardo. *Perspectivismo e multinaturalismo na América indígena*. Sao Paulo: PUC-RJ, 2002.

Walsh, Catherine. *Pedagogías Decoloniales. Prácticas insurgentes de resistir, (re) existir y (re) vivir*. Quito: Abya Yala, 2013.

Chapter Six

Now That We Are Back to School . . . Pandemic, Environment, and Community Links

Norma Georgina Gutiérrez Serrano

The Benito Juárez primary school in San Andrés de la Cal, municipality of Tepoztlán, Morelos, was one of seventy state schools at this educational level returning to in-person classes on June 21, 2021, as a pilot school. The present discussion registers the experience of the community after one year and four months without presential classes due to the COVID-19 outbreak.

During the twentieth century and now in the new millennium the people of the municipality of Tepoztlán have been characterized by the defense of their territory regarding their way of life and reproduction. These facts include historical events related to *Zapatismo*, in the beginning of the twentieth century, to more recent struggles against large-scale e governmental projects that usually tend to disrupt the environment connection between the inhabitants and nature. The projects intend to "modernize" the place by the construction of golf courses, new highways, and chairlifts that would require the destruction of the Sierra del Tepozteco hillside. In order words, progress would directly affect aquifers and the fragile system of rainfed crops, directly destroying the habitat of local flora and fauna that the inhabitants depend to survive (Salazar 2014; Velázquez García 2008; Olivares and Jacoby 2017). Besides the environmental problems, there are also cultural implications related to the mythical ancestral landscape that has sheltered the Tlahuica and mestizo cultures in the region for centuries. Another important fact interconnected to the community is the schools of the regions.

As already suggested, the identity of this community is basically rooted in ancestral ways of working the land and ways of life based on the defense of their land, their customs, and the culture of the region (Haraway 2019). The community life is very attached to the school system. The school is mostly directed to teach the importance of the community life that includes care for the natural environment. This is all expressed in multiple manifestations of everyday community life. With the spread of COVID-19, the community was deeply affected not only in health terms but also the collective ways of life.

Therefore, the present discussion is to analyze the impact of COVID-19 at the school system. The school is a representation of how *campesino* community life manifests itself. Besides the agricultural work, the students from the community dedicate themselves to latticework. Regarding agricultural systems, they have reproduced over centuries ancestral ways of planting and harvesting as well the commercialization of forest products. The entire process also includes inhabitants related to migratory system. Usually, they work temporally in Canada and the United States. Within this context, the return to school was buoyed up by the existence of this latticework—as a social safety net—that enabled the return of the children to school. Both the school and its educational project somehow relied on this communal "safety net" established over the years and renewed when the pandemic threatened "social normalcy." The continuation of programs and teaching efforts was possible due to the relationships with parents, townspeople, authorities, and even with migrants from this Tepoztec community.

Like in the rest of the country, the community of San Andrés de la Cal and its elementary schools, among them the Benito Juárez primary school, suspended activities for almost eighteen months, even without any COVID cases. The first cases were recorded in legal migrants (*golondrinos*) who work in the United States and Canada for short periods of time. Agricultural workers came back sick. Then the elderly population was the first to get it, and it was in that group that the first COVID deaths occurred among the population. At different times, school teachers got COVID, as did their families. However, none of the teachers live right in San Andrés.

This study gives us a large view of how the pandemic situation affected one of the many small rural communities, especially when activities started up again.

Rural education in Mexico and in Latin America is one of the most unfavorable sectors in society. Usually, they get less attention from public policy and educational research. However, this is a type of education that takes place in community spaces, where sustainable productive practices are preserved and the ways of life are closely linked to cultural traditions and maintained. At the same time, these ways of life interact with contemporary urban culture. Perhaps for these reasons, and because of everyday life outdoors, it recorded the lowest COVID indices in the country (because of urban information regarding the disease).

Thoughts about these experiences were a core interest in studying, especially, the return to school. This study shows how the school community came together and the prevalence of subtle forms of relationships and of learning process related to campesino children that went into action by creating a sort of network composed by teachers, students, and administrative staff. They made efforts to keep up educational system functioning during the pandemic. According to Daniel Bertaux in *Relatos de vida. Perspectiva etnosociológica*, under certain circumstances, to facilitate the process of communication between the teachers and the students, oral accounts and draws can be used by the teachers (Bertaux 2005). Yet words and different text formats are ways of getting closer to the underlying experiences and relationships (Contreras 2009). In writing this text, I use a personal narrative with aspects of self-ethnographic writing by means of which I show the conditions generating this text and the opportunity for working and talking with students when they returned to classes.

DESCRIBING SAN ANDRÉS DE LA CAL COMMUNITY IN TEPOZTLÁN, MORELOS

Tepoztlán is a municipality in the state of Morelos in Mexico. It is located on the slopes and hillside of the Tepoztec sierra, a mountainous chain with rocky terrain, copper-hued in the winter and exuberant green in summer. Its original population spoke the Nahuatl language and is known to have descended from the Tlahuica peoples. In the sixteenth century, Dominican monks built a convent and concentrated the peoples of the region around it on the slopes of the Tepoztec mountain, whose peak pre-Colombian features remain.

It is a rural community characterized by predominantly agricultural and forestry activities. The irregular orography of the region's soil prevents extensive use of tractors to harvest single-crop production and limits the use of technological packages of fertilizers. Inhabitants plant corn (maize) on rocky soil using a long dibble, or *coa*, as they walk through the fields. With this type of planting, they can succeed in attain a variegated form of co-growth crops. The family and the rest of the community are involved in this task: collective slashing and clearing, ploughing the field at least twice, before planting. These collective activities with seeds and earth, in the sun and outdoors, bring the community together in caring for the environment (Vega , Martínez-Bujan, and Paredes 2018). Thus, agroforestry activities are preserved and recreated by the cultural traditions of the peoples of the region since the 1940s, having combined with other forms of sustenance and employment.

San Andrés de la Cal is a small Tepoztec community located on the road from Cuernavaca, capital of the state of Morelos, to the municipality of Tepoztlán in the same state. With a population of more than a thousand inhabitants, it has the same productive characteristics as the entire municipality of Tepoztlán, with a distinctive feature of greater planting activity through the family organization, and strong ties to tradition and festivities related to the *milpa* (cornfield). It has sustainable agriculture, combining crops such as corn, beans, squash, tomatoes, chili peppers, and aromatic herbs such as *epazote* (Jesuit's tea). Such crops have permitted subsisting and providing the basic food basket for communities like these all over Mexico. Children from the community of San Andrés participate in the traditional ways of their parents. They take on activities related to crops and to caring for and feeding animals, according to their age, in addition to having playtime activities and family togetherness in the fields where campesinos typically work. Tepotztec children learn from their grandparents to choose, classify, and store seed, distinguishing creole seed from hybrid, and take care of farmyard animals. They know about seasonal cycles and follow cultural traditions regarding planting and sowing (Gutiérrez 2009; 2016). Therefore, children participate in community and environmental aspects, recreating community life in the field, in town, and in school. In past decades, subsistence activities in the region have combined with other commercial and job opportunities linked to the contemporary economy, including political and legal shifts in landholdings and, with it, the possibility of selling and privatizing communal *ejido* landholdings, therefore losing crop lands. This is one of the ways in which modernity leads to the dismantling of community agricultural and forestry activities.

In the rural life of San Andrés, the first COVID wave arrived late. Deaths during the first wave did not even amount to half a dozen. The first contagions were in families with migrant workers and with family members working in the city of Cuernavaca or in the domestic service of weekend houses of people regularly living in Mexico City. Some San Andrés inhabitants, who lost their jobs as workers or employees of companies in Cuernavaca or Mexico City, opted for returning to the fields, planting crops and raising animals. By doing this, they thought that they would get something to eat and didn't run the risk of getting sick.

According to Juanita Bermudez, they were in the fields and in the streets of the town, with no distance between them and no facemasks in the fields. Therefore, infections started because they held fiestas for the town's patron saints in December 2020 and January 2021. From them, many got infected. Yet, the municipality of Tepoztlán organized food drives, got products, organized producers from the towns, and, once a week, brought vegetables, beans, and corn to the families most isolated. They got lots of help, and there was enough food in town. Some had no work, but, in the fields, you could get work, tilling the soil then sowing and harvesting during the pandemic. What they couldn't recoup was the sale of handicrafts and cotton fabrics in the main square of Tepoztlán on Sundays.

THE ROLE OF BENITO JUÁREZ PRIMARY SCHOOL

The state of Morelos has 832 public primary schools,[1] fourteen of which are in the municipality of Tepoztlán. For the return to classes, after confinement due to the COVID-19 pandemic, two schools were selected by authorities to act as pilot schools. The first primary school, Santiago, adopted the modality of tutorials, by means of which children individually came to their teachers with questions. In San Andrés de la Cal, the primary school adopted an in-person modality, with a project consisting of pupils attending during school hours of 8 am to 12:30 pm, divided into two two-hour shifts, with a half hour for recess and changing shifts.

This school has a student population of 148, divided into six grades. The educational staff consists of a principal and six classroom teachers, one for each year. Classes also receive the attention of one physical education teacher and an English teacher, in addition to having a volunteer art teacher from the Waldorf school who lives in the community and provides support with therapeutic art techniques once a week for each classroom.

Its importance goes back to the 1940 as well as the Revolutionary era, when the school occupied a small space next to one of the two Catholic churches. The townspeople themselves built the first schoolrooms, which still exist despite the damage the school underwent in the 2017 earthquake. The official registry of the school, with the name of Mexican President Benito Juárez, as well as expanded classroom space, date back to the 1970s, as confirmed by the present principal. The school reproduced community life as well as its historically important commitment to the environment. Rural education took a serious pounding once the nationalist model became exhausted and modernization and the model of global economy was given entry. Rural teachers' training was abandoned financially and later hit straight on (Ronquillo 2018).

The last political action severely punishing teacher training throughout the country was the educational reforms at the end of the first decade of the twentieth century. They set their sights on international standards of evaluation and quality. The direct emphasis was on individual performance and quantifiable results, to the detriment of community relationships and forms of collective learning, of collaboration and exchange, which was the basis for organizing work in a rural community. For several decades, rural education provided training for future rural teachers. San Andrés was known as a town of teachers. Up until recent years, this also made it a base for training professionals. By the year 2010, many homes had members with professional degrees: lawyers, operational technicians, accountants, historians. As modernity and supposed development projects went forward, basic education in the municipality of Tepoztlán and the state of Morelos barely allowed their inhabitants to obtain a certificate to work as chauffeurs, stevedores at central markets, waitresses, cashiers, or cooks in city establishments. A deterioration of educational credentials at a basic level grew according to how the economic crises of capital ebbed and flowed. Even so, for almost four decades, the neoliberal federal government decided to strengthen an educational model based on competencies, on individual performance, and on a quality of education measured and quantified according to international standards, foreign to the capacities and response-abilities[2] of agricultural communities.

As a result of educational reforms, rural schools have been modifying their original sense of being. For example, they have begun to change their teaching staffs, receiving teachers with a variety of training, but without having studies at rural normal schools. One example of this is the school at San Andrés. Teachers that have been teaching at this school for the past twelve years said they try to maintain a close relationship with planting crops in the region, even owning land and working it. The newer teaching staff leads a more urban lifestyle. One of the teachers is the daughter of a doctor in Tepoztlán.[3] The principal, Lupita Sndoval, has held her position for four years and lives in the nearby city of Cuernavaca. The rest of the teaching staff lives in the municipality of Tepoztlán or close to it: two teachers in Yecapixtla, another two in Yautepec, one more in Cuautla, and the rest in the municipal head of Tepoztlán.

Despite the new makeup of the teaching staff at this school, even now, the strength of ties to the community culture are maintained and they manage to embrace and imbue the primary school with these types of with these types of land-based connections. The 2008 socio-demographic census done in the locality of San Andrés showed strong activity related to agricultural and forestry production among area households, with a notable combination of providing domestic services, gardening, local commerce, tourism, food sales, transportation services, professional employees, and independent professionals. In addition, there is also the financial tradition of migrating to the United States and Canada that dates back to the 1940s. There is legal migration for six months maximum per year. Therefore, the population has a variety of income and financial sustenance. This corresponds to 2017 data provided by Municipal Diagnostics of Tepoztlán.

In the accounts of children and adults from the community taken between 2008 and 2010, there was constant talk about shared activities in agriculture or herding within the family dynamics of the households of this agricultural community. The ongoing legal migration of parents to the United States and Canada supposes the active participation of grandparents in caring for the children. They too are committed to defending he environment of their territory (Castañeda and Corral 2015). In these everyday means of family production, children learn to relate to the family and the overall environment of its livelihood, as well as to productive work in the fields (Robles 2012). It is in this everyday life where social learning takes place, which, according to Etiene Wenger (2001), is at the core of human existence.

During the pandemic, a good number of the migrant workers returned home and some of them came back sick. Other migrants postponed their return. They managed to stay in the north of the continent during the worst months of the pandemic, not returning until almost the end of May 2021. Families in the community have become accustomed to living with the absence of parents, siblings, or other members of the family since the 1940s.

A PILOT PROJECT FOR RETURNING TO CLASSES: MOBILIZATION OF RELATIONS IN NETWORK[4]

In Mexico, after the CanSino vaccine was provided to teachers in the national educational system, a return to classes was announced in June 2021 for the basic level of this system once several states had reached a health-warning green "traffic" light. In the case of the state of Morelos, in the month of July 2021, different municipalities returned to classes through a system of opening seventy pilot schools. It was done differently by each school and municipality. As I stated earlier, in the case of the municipality of Tepoztlán, two schools participated in the program: one of them, the Benito Juárez school in San Andrés de la Cal.

The functioning of the pilot school at San Andrés was based on a series of agreements and negotiations among authorities, the principal and supervisor, and teachers from that school. This expressed local forms of relationships with diverse social and community actors.

The official recommendation was to open with half the students from each room and alternate the group attending each day, for the full day. However, activities were to be done without pauses, recess, or meals during the school day.

In light of this, the principal organized the school by what was called the Pilot Project, adjustments or definitions being made together with the school's teachers and possibilities for students to do homework. According to M. Rios, a teacher,

> If, for us, it's hard to sit still for four hours, for the children, even more. So, the teachers' idea was, in the first two hours, to receive one part of the students from every classroom and, in the next two hours, the other students, all on the same day.
>
> No parents were to come in. They don't eat here, nor take recess.
>
> Teacher participation is voluntary. I talked a lot with them. The decision was in their hands. Fortunately, they consented. It's something needed by the children, the parents, the teachers themselves, the school, the community.
>
> I told parents we were trying, but unsure about the opening date of the school. The idea is to start in two weeks, but we can't guarantee. May it'll be in a week or a day. It could be two or even more. We asked for their understanding . . .
>
> This is a project, an attempt, likewise, for what we can do for the next school year. (June 21, 2021)

Ulloa López, another teacher, declared that:

> One idea was to divide them up by last name, alphabetically. But, when someone isn't here, in communities like this, you forget at times inhabitants have the same last names. Here, the majority are Benítez or Bermúdez. So, other criteria were used, according to teachers' considerations. (López, June 21, 2021)

Besides the dynamic nature of the ties in this educational community and agreements and negotiations in the networks in this brief return to school, we also observed the extension of school ties beyond its physical and geographic limits. The closing of the school year for those in sixth grade supposed a simple graduation ceremony, with the election of the respective class sponsors. In this case, a Morelos migrant to the United States sponsored the graduating class and sent presents to each of the graduates.

INTERNET EXPERIENCES

During the COVID-19 pandemic, the San Andrés de la Cal primary school, just like the rest of the schools in the country and those of many other countries, faced the challenge of shifting educational attention to virtual scenarios. In the case at hand, transfer was not immediate. In the rural milieu of Tepoztlán, families could count on electronic means and internet, even though they might not have been sufficient for simultaneous use by household members. However, despite having the equipment, telephone, and internet, signals could be rather unstable due to its orography. This situation favored the first educational option being mixed in nature during the pandemic.

At the San Andrés school, teachers began by sending homework in student notebooks while the health-warning system in the locality in 2020 was coded as a green, yellow, or orange "traffic" light. Teachers attended school each Friday and checked the exercises they had previously given out in students' notebooks. This way of dealing with the situation was combined with setting up WhatsApp groups, though not all students managed to connect or keep up with communications.

According to Lupita Sandoval,

Parents left backpacks with children's notebooks. They even left them with the school watchman. Teachers arrived on Friday and checked the work and left other exercises, and that's how we were, outside in the schoolyard and without parents coming in. . . . At that time, I tried to attend to first graders one day a week in the patio and sixth graders the same, once a week in the schoolyard. I was worried about these two grades, how some came and how the others were going to go . . . later, when the health-warning system was red, the same parents started to ask to be attended virtually. One of the first-grade teachers was doing so and they wanted to . . . so, in January of this year, they started to attend to them on Zoom or Meet. (Lupita Sandoval 2021).

As already mentioned, during these times, one frequently used technological support was exchanging messages through WhatsApp between teachers and students. Videos were also shared to support the teaching. Occasionally, there were videos for the parents themselves, to help in the process.

According to A. Silva,

My wife filmed me solving math problems and I sent them to the parents, so they would know how to solve what I was asking the children to do. I also made videos with the book open. Those were for the children. (teacher A. Silva, June 28, 2021)

In January I started to attend the children on Zoom two hours, two and a half hours, every third day. This was when we could no longer come to school, when the health-warning system was red. First, there were 26 children I had connected up with on Zoom, but slowly they started to disconnect. I ended up with seventeen . . . they got tired and started saying they had to go eat or were hungry. (sixth-grade teacher, A. Silva, June 28, 2021)

I split the class into six groups of four pupils each. I attended them for one hour on Zoom, since, with more than one hour, I started to see them putting their feet on the table or desk, turning around, getting up. More than an hour was hard because I gave them math . . . despite that, I now realize that the division they were already solving well or, at least, they tuned into me, because I don't know

if maybe the parents did them, or some of them didn't remember how. Today
I had to sit down with several of them to solve problems. (teacher, A. Silva,
June 28, 2021)

Sometimes I received homework at 10 at night, even Saturdays and Sundays,
though I answered them during the week and daytime. (teacher, V. Peñaloza,
June 28, 2021)

Another teacher named Lupita added that:

What happened was that parents could only help their children when they
returned home from work.
   On April 30, we called up each class to the patio to give them small gifts. I
saw they[5] were really serious. They seemed depressed, my daughter said.

In these short accounts by teachers, we can see a variety of dynamic, spontaneous, and creative actions taken on the part of the school and teachers
to tackle the suspension of student attendance due to the pandemic. Each
teacher initiated different ways of directly relating to their class within the
institutional framework, while, in general, they were also adapting. Ways of
teaching and interaction were modified, including the intervention of parents
and even relatives of the teachers themselves. Forms of relationship were
activated. We might say that relations of the school community were dynamic
and, spontaneously, they managed to take the educational steps needed.
   The consequences of ways of dealing with education supposed that routines
at home, at work, and during school activities were out of sync. This called
for constant adaptation to maintain contact and a rhythm of schoolwork.

TOOLS FOR QUESTIONING AND
REFLECTIONS ON THE ENCOUNTERS

My own presence and brief moments attending the classes related to the pilot
project during the first two weeks gave rise to important exchanges among
students, teachers, the principal, and the school-zone supervisor. Without
any possibility of foreseeing the extent of these encounters and exchanges,
I started to evaluating teachers' pedagogical efforts during the suspension
of the activities due to the pandemic, as well as their efforts to encourage
children's written and pictorial expressions related to their return to classes.
   I continued my short chats with four teachers, the principal, and the supervisor during the interval student activities. From these exchanges, these data
provided me with an understanding of how the educational system attended

the students while classes were suspended and when they returned to school. In addition, I also paid attention to the teachers' performance and impressions after coming back.

With a few exercises to encourage students to write, I began to study their reflections on their return to classes and self-perception on pandemic times within the school context.

According to Larrosa, in his book, *Alteridad en educación* (2009), "the subject of learning is the subject of experience."

> La experiencia, ante todo, es un paso, un pasaje, una estancia. Si la palabra experiencia contiene el ex de lo que está fuera, también tiene ese perse que es un radical indoeuropeo para las palabras que tienen que ver con el viaje, con el paso, con el camino, con el viaje. La experiencia supone, pues, salir de uno mismo hacia otra cosa. (Larrosa 2009, 17)

Experience, first of all, is a step, a passage, a sojourn. If the word experience contains the ex of what is outside, it likewise has that perse which is an Indo-European radical for words having to do with voyage, with passage, with pathway, with journey. Experience therefore supposes going out from oneself toward something else.

To achieve answers of a collective nature, I suggested an ongoing writing experience starting from sentences in the plural, as triggers for the children's narratives. Therefore, I proposed the following open-ended sentence: "Now that we are back to school . . . "

I also proposed an ongoing or collective text. Each child was to write phrases or sentences about the trigger sentence which would then be read by another colleague by adding additional narratives to the previous texts. The intention was to generate a sort of narrative latticework.

According to Larrosa, "la reflexividad imprime un movimiento desde adentro, desde la subjetividad hacia su ubicación afuera. En este caso, el exterior supondría la situación en la escuela de los alumnos/ reflexivity imprints a movement from inside, from subjectivity toward its location outside. In this case, the *outside* would suppose the situation at the students' school." Based on these principles, I tried to link personal experience to a collective reflexivity. The ongoing writing exercise created a stir in the pupils. They looked about uneasily and gave disguised smiles to those to whom they passed the sheet of paper containing the previous narrative. They read them attentively. There were some that started writing right away, others remained quiet a bit, while others showed bewilderment and let me help them. The exchange of ideas between two or three younger ones was another spontaneous strategy among younger pupils, serving as support for all.

Although the exercises attempted to delve into the students' experience of returning to class in a pandemic situation, it is possible to recognize that in doing these exercises, there is the generation of another experience represented by the exteriorization of the reflexivity regarding relationships and exchanges. From this perspective, the format proposed for the exercises was set up so it could generate experiences of a collective nature.

What the students showed from their experience was their relationship with the educational situation, that is, school, teachers, and classmates, during times of pandemic and during the return to classes.

Student writings showed lively expressions about returning, a sort of growing commitment to be back in school. Written accounts seemed to mirror adult opinions, perhaps familiar to them, about the relevance of being in school and studying. They reflected a future image of their personal development. In total, eighteen continuous accounts were collected from the subgroupings of students belonging to the last three primary grades. In these sentences that each child added to, there were repeated expressions such as:

It is noteworthy that among these expressions were ideas about commitment, compliance with the norms, and school or family discipline, much more than those related to a desire to play or spend time with classmates. Perhaps such a position is a way of wanting to contribute to the reopening of their school from the viewpoint of adults. Nor did such a position hamper expressing their looking forward to getting together, reestablishing activities related to everyday exchanges between students, or even beyond school walls.

Table 6.1.

Expressions Written by Fourth, Fifth, and Sixth Graders	Frequency
Be a good person	16
Be a better person	
Let's work/study a lot	10
We'll pay attention to the teacher and we'll obey	10
We'll study everything teachers teach us	8
I'll get up early	8
We'll get there on time	4
We'll play football when we get out	3
We'll all go home together with my dog	3
We'l play Super Rider (videogame)	2
We'll hug and talk	2
We're not going to fight	1
I'm going to bring gum for my friends	1
Let's draw Zaida (videogame)	1
I'll go with my classmates to play in the caves (area outside school)	1
I'm going to ride around on a bike with my friends	1

ON RETURN TO THE RESEARCH SCENARIO:
A VIEW TOWARD THE EXPERIENCE ITSELF

This text resulted from the initial interest and concern of maintaining contact with the school community of San Andrés during times of confinement due to the COVID-19 pandemic. At the end of 2019, the first exchanges began in a basic education research project at rural schools in Brazil and Mexico, which we called Letters without Borders (*Cartas sin fronteras*). The difficulties imposed by suspended school attendance put any possibility of the project on pause. In this situation, the school principal and I kept up friendly contact, sharing concerns and uncertainties on the course of the pandemic and the situation of school suspension we were in.

My contact with the San Andrés primary school began in 2008, when I began a research project at the school, along with the participation of other colleagues and graduate students. This work was linked to other projects, our own and those of other colleagues the research center and at the Universidad Nacional Autónoma de México. This led me to expand my relationship with the Benito Juárez school and the community to more than twelve years. Even though the school, students, and teaching actors changed over the years, my relationship with the school and the community were kept up through renewed ties. In all this, one relevant influence, undoubtedly, was the edition of materials on the school and community with the editorial backing of the Universidad Nacional Autónoma de México.

Therefore, I was able to find a friendly community environment and an open school community receptive to my return, notwithstanding changes in authorities and in the educational policy.

BETWEEN SILENCE AND OBSERVATION TO
REINSERT ONESELF INTO THE DIALOGUE

"Generally speaking, this group is quiet. They don't participate much" (sixth-grade teacher).

There were also other groups of students that did not participate like others. According to Mr. Silva,

Es que nosotros mismos no tenemos claro pedagógicamente qué hacer. . . . Empecé, estas dos semanas, con temas nuevos. Decidí trabajar en proyectos para llamar su atención nuevamente. Por ejemplo, sobre el tema del movimiento de la luna y la tierra, y se animaron e hicieron preguntas después del video. (Professor A. Silva, June 28, 2021)

It's just we ourselves aren't clear pedagogically about what to do. . . . I began, these two weeks, with new topics. I decided to work on projects to get their attention again. For example, on the topic of the movement of the moon and the Earth, and they perked up and asked questions after the video.

Los veo felices de venir. Creo que prefieren venir, ya que los padres se cansan y se desesperan. Ya que, aun siendo un maestro teniendo preparación, si alguien, como un padre, se desespera al tratar de enseñar a sus hijos, no está capacitado para eso. Creo que deben pasar algunos malos momentos, mal genio de sus padres, y venir a la escuela ya que les gusta más que quedarse en casa. Además, creo que es como volver por ellos, ¿cómo explicarlo? Pues sí, como una esperanza de que las cosas vuelvan a ser como antes. prefieren venir. (Professor A. Silva, June 28, 2021)

I see them happy to come. I think they prefer coming, since parents get tired and desperate. Since, even as a teacher having preparation, if someone, like a parent, gets desperate when trying to teach their children, they aren´t trained for that. I think they must pass some bad moments, ill temper in their parents, and come to school since they like it better than staying at home. Besides, I think it´s like returning for them, how can I explain it? Well, yes, like a hope that things return to be as before. They prefer to come.

Lo importante para mí es el vínculo entre el maestro y los niños. Eso es lo que nos deja trabajar. Ya habíamos trabajado juntos antes de la pandemia y después con videos y Zoom. Supongo que eso me ayuda a mantenerlos atentos y participativos. Hay algunos que siempre hablan y están inquietos, pero hacen el trabajo. La interacción social es fundamental para los niños. Bueno, hay un caso. Un niño con un defecto del habla volvió a aislarse. Solo hablaba con los que conocía y, antes de la pandemia, su interacción con los demás había aumentado y, ahora, se calla y se aísla del resto. (Professor A. Silva, June 28, 2021)

What's important for me is the link between the teacher and the children. That's what lets us work. We had already worked together before the pandemic and later with videos and Zoom. I suppose that helps me keep them attentive and participating. There are some who always talk and are fidgety, but they do the work. Social interaction is fundamental for children. Well, there is one case. A boy with a speech defect went back to isolating himself. He only talked to those he knew and, before the pandemic, his interaction with others had increased and, now, he keeps quiet and isolates himself from the rest.

According to the teacher L. Sandoval,

A las maestras se les decía mucho sobre atender el lado emocional de los niños, escucharlos, animarlos a hablar. . . . Ahora, eso era lo más importante. (L. Sandoval, June 23, 2021)

A lot was said to the teachers about attending to the emotional side of the children, listening to them, encouraging them to talk. . . . Now, that was what was most important.

All of these accounts express the teachers' perception of a change in the children's attitudes upon their return after the pandemic. In general, students were more silent, inactive, and participated less, as the teachers stated. Even the possibility of depressive behavior was considered. This clear change in the students' behavior was perceived for more than one year of isolation. Students, their relatives, and the rest of their community endured together similar patterns of behavior. However, it might be worthwhile to consider that the school community is basically formed by rural indigenous children. To that end, Ruth Paradise's (2010) ethnographic study allows us to see a reinterpretation of the types of relationships and learning in Indian children. Previous studies related to social learning such as those by Wenger (2001) and Paradise (2010) reinforce that the social learning takes place according to the children's situation and cultural context. In the case of Paradise, he emphasizes that this kind of interaction between community and affiliates is typical among indigenous communities. In those communities, family interaction and individual ties are mutually reinforced. These practices are accompanied by productive family practices that are reinforced.

One might consider that, during the time spent at home, the forms of relationship with family and the forms of community existence, including the organization of family agricultural work (Robles 2012), came to take up more space within the everyday dynamics of the children, who returned to the school scenario cautiously. The same caution was perceived by a student and myself between 2008 and 2010 (Camerán 2011) in this same school community: children observed the activities, silently and initially timidly, and gradually opened up to participation once it was proposed they express themselves through drawing and participating in storytelling. This was a dynamic very appreciated among them.

Taking these forms of tacit collaboration among children in agricultural communities into consideration is probably the best way to interact with them when returning to school. This method was introduced within school pedagogy for consideration, and it was recognized as another way of understanding and interacting with children who belong to rural spaces. Therefore, the method allowed better understanding of the community experience in which these children are growing and developing.

FINAL REFLECTIONS

The COVID-19 pandemic reached the community of San Andrés slowly and later when compared to urban communities. Initially, there were only a few deaths and the rates of contagion did not rise notably until the end of 2021. Agricultural and rural activities were, for some inhabitants, a way to continue working outdoors and with physical distancing. The town reported a loss of jobs and commerce, but they continued and even increased agricultural activities.

In order to solve the school problems regarding the presential attendance of children at San Andrés school, administrative staff and teachers told me how they tried to overcome the problem during the pandemic. Inhabitants of the community, and also entire families, and not only parents, supported the efforts of students and teachers. Another important step in the process was the role of municipal authorities in order to adapt the school curricula to the material conditions. After coming back to school, teachers quickly enlisted previous ties to parents, municipal authorities, the other inhabitants of San Andrés, and even migrants from up north.

In this approach to school during the pandemic, I was able to better identify the complex and broad-ranging school and community network constantly being woven by administrators, teachers, children, and parents at the Benito Juárez School. Trying out and developing new forms of relationship between teachers and the students was relatively easier because of the virtual communication or distance learning model.

In the continuous writing exercise, students showed interest in returning to classes by adhering to school normativity and the future horizon, casting aside their interests and enthusiasm for getting back together with classmates.

I spent two weeks at their school, and I realized that the project was successful, especially for depending on community support. Community relationships were possible because they had the support of teachers, who evince efforts to sustain learning, keeping the school in tune with the community's way of productive life. They embraced them as participants in their festivities and foodstuffs, integrating them into community life. From this point of view, it was the school atmosphere that was the beneficiary of the community relationship. Perhaps the strongest reflection left to me with was the necessity to understand the forms of relationship after classes were suspended due to COVID-19.

The school's teachers highly value the interaction among students to learn.

After returning to the classes, teachers were surprised with the student responses. Their silence was a prevailing attitude after their return to classes.

Observing and studying the forms of community relations might help teachers and school administrators to better understand the students' attitude.

At first, the sense of isolation, indifference, and silence from the students was a common attitude. Therefore, social learning skills were used in order to overcome the barriers of communication. Moreover, if teachers and school authorities see themselves within the larger latticework of the community, and not only as educational professionals, they will be able to continue with the support they need to work and, from there, continue strengthening an educational project of a community nature beyond the educational models imposed by dominant Western culture, which tends toward individualization, separation, and distancing from collective forms of production and strong links to the environment. The reflection that is the product of this text also allowed me to observe myself and consider myself part of this network.

Finally, I would like to reinforce that the forms of relationship of the school community are expressions of the community's strength ties through which the individuals organize means of political resistance not only the preservation of natural environment but also recreation and constant revitalization of a culture woven into the everyday life of tilling the soil and of sharing experiences.

INTERVIEWS

(June 21–23, 2021) Interviews with teacher Lupita Sandoval, school principal, done by Norma Georgina Gutiérrez Serrano, at the Benito Juárez de San Andrés de la Cal primary school.

(June 22, 2021) Personal conversation with teacher Mario López, zone supervisor, at the Benito Juárez de San Andrés de la Cal primary school.

(June 28–30, 2021) Interview with teacher Lupita Sandoval, done by Norma Georgina Gutiérrez Serrano, at the Benito Juárez de San Andrés de la Cal primary school.

(June 29, 2021) Personal conversation with teacher Rosaura Ponce, at the Benito Juárez de San Andrés de la Cal primary school.

(June 30, 2021) Personal conversation with teacher Victoria Peñaloza, at the Benito Juárez de San Andrés de la Cal primary school.

(June 30, 2021) Interviews with fourth-grade teacher Antonio Silva, done by Norma Georgina Gutiérrez Serrano, at the Benito Juárez de San Andrés de la Cal primary school.

(June 30, 2021) Personal conversation with teacher Aida González, art therapist, at the Benito Juárez de San Andrés de la Cal primary school.

(February 15, 2022) Personal conversation with Antonia Bermudez in San Adnrés de la Cal.

NOTES

1. Secretaría de Educación Pública, Dirección General de Planeación, Programación y Estadística Educativa. Estadística Educativa, Morelos 2018–2019. http://planeacion.sep.gob.mx/Doc/estadistica_e_indicadores/estadistica_e_indicadores_entidad_federativa/estadistica_e_indicadores_educativos_17MOR.pdf
2. Term modified by Donna Haraway, 2019.
3. Information obtained from the 2008 socio-demographic census (Gutiérrez 2009).
4. In this text, I use the notion of community ties and linkage as forms of essential relationships in the town of Tepoztlán and the notion of networking in relation to the actions generated by the San Andrés primary school to attain, maintain, generate, and coproduce relationships with the community.
5. April 30 is the Children's Day date in Mexico.

REFERENCES

Anderson, Leon., "Analytic Autoethnography." *Journal of Contemporary Ethnography* 35, no. 4 (2006): 373–95.
Bertaux, Daniel. *Relatos de vida. Perspectiva etnosociológica.* Spain: SGU, 2005.
Camerán, Erica. "Experiencias siguiendo las huellas de la pedagogía deloprimido." Doctoral thesis, Universidad de Bolonia, 2011.
Castañeda, Intandihui, and Carolina Corral. *Documental: La batalla de las cacerolas.* Mexico: Sandía digital, 2015. https://www.youtube.com/watch?v=yxzgOvRPeZA&ab_channel=CarolinaCorral
Contreras, José. "Prologue." In *Alteridad en educación* (Argentina: FLACSO, 2009).
Gutiérrez, Norma G. "Relatos de la vida productiva alrededor del maíz. Cultura, conocimiento y aprendizaje." In *Cultura y representaciones sociales* 4, no. 7 (2009).
Gutiérrez, Norma G. *En San Andrés Tnextila sembramos maíz.* Mexico: UNAM-CRIM, 2016).
Haraway, Donna. *Seguir con el problema. Generar parentesco en el Chthuluceno.* Mexico: Consonni, 2019.
Larrosa, Jorge. "Alteridad en educación." *Alteridad en educación* (2009): 13–44.

Paradise, Ruth. "La interacción mazahua en su contexto cultural: ¿pasividad o colaboración tácita?" In *Socialización, lenguajes y culturas infantiles: Estudios interdisciplinarios*, edited by L. de León, 77–94. Mexico: CIESAS, 2010.

Rangel, Alfonso. "La educación rural mexicana y la educación fundamental en el inicio del CREFAL." *Revista Interamericana de Educación de Adultos* 28, no. 2 (2006): 169–76.

Robles, Adriana. "Participación de niños indígenas mazahuas en la organización familiar del trabajo." *Working Papers on Culture, Education and Human Development* no. 8 (2012).

Ronquillo, Víctor. *Ayotzinapa: la otra historia*. México: Universidad Iberoamericana, 2018.

Salazar, Ana María. *Tepoztlán. Movimiento etnopolítico y patrimonio cultural. Una batalla victoriosa ante el poder global*. Mexico: UNAM-IIA, 2014.

Skiliar, Carlos, and Jorge Larrosa. *Alteridad en educación*. Argentina: FLACSO, 2009.

Vega, Cristina, Raquel Martínez-Bujan, and Miriam Paredes. *Experiencias y vínculos cooperativos en el sostenimiento de la vida en América Latina y el sur de Europa*. Madrid: Traficantes de sueños, 2018.

Velázquez García, Mario Alberto. "La construcción de un movimiento ambiental en México: El club de golf en Tepoztlán, Morelos." *Región y sociedad* XXN (2008): 43.

Wenger, Etiene. *Comunidades en práctica: Aprendizaje, significado e identidad*. Argentina: Paidos, 2001.

PROCESS AND INQUIRY TOOLS

Bruner, Jerome. *La Fábrica de historias*. Mexico: Fondo de Cultura Económica, 2013.

Clandinin, Jean, and Michael Connelly. *Narrative Inquiry: Experience and Story in Qualitative Research*. San Francisco, CA: Jossey-Bass, 2000.

Connelly, M., and Jean Clandinin. "Relatos de experiencia e investigación narrativa." In *Déjame que te cuente: Ensayos sobre narrativa y educación*, edited by Jorge Larrosa, Remei Arnaus, Virginia Ferrer, Nuria Pérez De Lara, and Maxine Greene, 11–59. Barcelona: Laertes, 1995.

Contreras, J., and Nuria Pérez. *Investigar la experiencia educativa*. Madrid: Morata, 2010.

Olivares, José, and Jacob Jacoby. "Tepoztlán's Highway to Nowhere." *Nacla reporting on the Americas since 1967*, November 30, 2017.

Chapter Seven

Chronicle of Life during the COVID-19 Pandemic in Mexico

Georgina Vega Fregoso

Since March 2020, the Mexican government through National Health Day recognized that COVID-19 was a *force majeure*. As a result, it paralyzed daily acitivites around the country. This fact instigated me to ask about the relationship between pandemics and the health of the ecosystems and how healthcare is understood in the nature versus culture relationship. As an anthropologist, I will discuss my personal experience and adaptation related to the social changes at the onset of the pandemic. Here, I will take into consideration the holistic perspective to understand humans' fragile conditon as well the human relationship with the ecosystem.

This text is a narrative construction that willl allow me to explain how I coped with my condition as a mother, researcher, and teacher during 2020 and how reality was woven into my life thread. By using autoethnograhy, I aim to provide means of understanding reality and the emotional experience that surrounded the events. Emotions were particularly important to the process. According to Burns, "emotions, in particular, are fertile ground for making a narrative impressive" (Burns 2019, 198). This writing emerges from my experience, and my purpose here is to reveal the dominant discourses and offer alternatives to understand the reality during and after the pandemic.

The methodological strategy started from the ethnographic register and the autoethnographic perspective, considering, as Mercedes Blanco argues, that the autoethnographic proposal is the indissoluble mixture between the dimensions traditionally called objective and subjective (Blanco 2012, 172). As I progressed in the experience, I recorded informal conversations, memes, photographs, and drawings. I generated a set of interviews related to how various subjects explained the reasons why the coronavirus emerged and its mechanisms of contagion. I also recorded diverse opinions about the public's handling of the pandemic and how it has changed the public's lives. While there is no definitive agreement on the boundaries of the self-ethnographic, I agree with Kirstin Koeltzsch, who points out that the present, the past, self-observation, and reflexivity are central categories in autoethnography in a perspective of thinking in present tense and how it happens on us or in our bodies (Koeltzsch 2021).

The selected facts in the present narrative are from March to December 2020; they demonstrate what it means to take care of one's health. I also took into consideration two competitive discourses (i.e, from a common citzen as well as from agents that belong to dominat sectors of society). Following Jonathan Wyatt and Toni E. Adams in their theorization of autoehtnography on the books *On (Writing) Families* (2014), I consider this narrative to be a part of the nation's collective history. I propose this work as a creative act in which writing is a kind of incarnation coupled with the possibility of making a story from our intimate history.

I will emphasize opinions and descriptions that were part of my experience with COVID-19 during the confinement. Researching the social imaginary around the pandemic allowed me to contrast fears, values, beliefs, and expectations regarding the risk of contracting the virus. It is also relevant, as Castoriadis highlights, to point out that the social imaginary is more than social representation; the social imaginary is the self-creation of society as such, power in the collective anonymity, so it is possible to capture the imaginaries and subjectivity of social actors through their creative expressions (Castoriadis 2005, 12).

GETTING TO KNOW SARS-COV-2

This story begins when I learned from Twitter, at the end of December 2019, that a group of patients with pneumonia of unknown etiology were reported at the city of Wuhan, China. A few weeks later, on February 11, it was announced that a new SARS-CoV-2, a type of coronavirus has isolated; the World Health Organization had named it "COVID-19." From this official date, a number of public narratives of the pandemic by SARS-CoV-2 emerged (Guarner 2020, 420). At that moment, I began to read the information available about the virus without imagining that the worst was about to come.

By reading the news, I came to know that the World Health Organization declared the disease a pandemic, specifically a flu pandemic of global reach, and part of the global populations had no immunity against this virus. According to Jeannette Guarner in the editorial "Three Emerging Coronaviruses in Two Decades: The Story of SARS, MERS, and Now

COVID-19" (Guarner 2020, 420) from the year 2000 we have witnessed several pandemics caused by three types of coronavirus that have produced public health outbreaks. Moreover, to Yvonne Xinyi Lim, the disease also had a zoonotic profile. Lim explains that "coronaviruses are enveloping, non-segmented, single-stranded, positive-sense RNA viruses" (Lim et al. 2016, 3). So far, seven coronaviruses have been identified as barriers causing disease in humans (zoonoses), carrying symptoms that go from mild respiratory infection to more serious pulmonary illnesses, such as the severe acute respiratory syndrome (SARS).

The types of coronaviruses that have caused these types of outbreaks, such as the one identified at that time in Wuhan, are SARS-CoV that first appeared at Guangdong, China, in 2003, followed by MERS-CoV that appeared on 2012 in the Middle East causing widespread respiratory disease. A complete genome sequencing and phylogenetic analysis, in March 2020, made it possible to classify the virus responsible for the COVID-19 pandemic as a coronavirus, of the betacoronavirus genus. The *Coronavirinae* subfamily that shares between 79 percent and 50 percent, respectively, of genomic similarity with SARS-CoV and MERS-CoV (Saltigeral-Simental and León-Lara 2020, 466).

I also discussed with my colleagues at the Academy of Environment and Health at the University of Guadalajara about the lethality of the COVID-19 and if Mexican federal government was prepared to deal with the problem. We knew that the only parameter the government had for crises management was related to the government's public health campaign to confront the dengue crises in 2019. It was in September 2019 that national newspapers had headlines such as: "Jalisco Stater urges to declare State urges to declare an epidemiological alert for dengue." In October 2019, the state of Jalisco had the highest mortality rate from dengue in Mexico.

In order to better understand the decision-making process at the national level, I began to look for analyses on specific characteristics of the virus SARS-CoV-2 in relation to SARS-CoV-1. I found that under experimental conditons, the observations by Doremalen, Bushmaker, and Morris were consistent with my expectations regarding the means of transmission as well as the epidemiological characteristics of the virus. The "differences in the epidemiological characteristics of these viruses probably arise from other factors, including high viral loads in the upper respiratory tract and the possibility that people infected with SARS-CoV-2 shed and transmit the virus while they are asymptomatic" (Doremalen, Bushmaker, and Morris 2020, 1564). At that point, I wondered about the relationship between environmental degradation and COVID-19. Among the causes of degradation in Mexico are changes in land use, urban sprawl, and intensive agriculture, all factors that affect human and non-human lives. I began to consider the degradation of ecosystems, food quality, and levels of marginalization and poverty, as well as epidemiological

characteristics of the Mexican population, as social and environmental determinants of health. So the poorest urban population without having the basic
necessities satisfied like adequate nutrition, health, education, and habitation
became one of the hardest hit by the COVID-19 pandemic (Ortiz-Hernández
and Pérez-Sastré 2020, 5).

On March 16, 2020, the first mandatory confinement and the suspension of face-to-face activities at the University de Guadalajara in Jalisco
was decreed. Faced with this scenario, federal authorities had to organize a
complex set of collective actions aimed at maintaining public health. A week
later, the federal government issued an invitation to house confinement. A
nationwide strategy of public health communication was launched. However,
accurate data on the forms of contagion was scarce, and the identification of
COVID-19 symptoms was still preliminary. Mandatory confinement was a
measure that sought to contribute to the protection of families. While it was
clear that absolute confinement was not an option for working-class families
in need of a basic income, in reality, full confinement was only possible fo
middle- and upper-class households.

PANDEMICS AND ECOSYSTEM HEALTH IN MEXICO

To understand the relationship between pandemic and ecosystem we must
know that, according to the WHO (World Health Organization) there are three
epidemiological conditions that compromise the health of the population:
outbreaks, epidemics, and pandemics. An outbreak is "the sudden appearance
of a disease due to an infection in a specific place and at a certain time" such
as poisoning and measles; an epidemic is "a disease that spreads actively
due to the fact that the outbreak gets out of control and continues over time,
increasing the number of cases in a specific geographical area," such is the
case of smallpox; and a pandemic, in turn, "affects more than one continent
and that the cases in each country are no longer imported but caused by community transmission" (Pulido 2020, 1). Such was the case in Mexico in April
2020. In the case of COVID-19, a disease that occurs in animals and that
can be transmitted to humans under natural conditions is called a zoonosis
(Villalobos 2016, 76).

Faced with the study of pandemics, at least two positions can be adopted.
The first may be an upward approach, that is, the one that emphasizes that
there are always more daily deaths than those reported in official records and
other documentary sources. Considering that, indeed, there is an underreporting of deaths (Villar 2018, 80). This approach emphasizes that deaths from
COVID-19 have been much more than those reported by Mexico's secretary
of health. The upward approach has been highly promoted by national news

media, even though journalists are not experts on public heath issues such like COVID-19. The offical reports state the downward perspective, which considers that there were not so many deaths caused only by the pandemic and that an important proportion of deaths can be attributed to other causes that are synergistic to the SARS-CoV-2 virus. In addition to the COVID-19 death records, other preexisting clinical, environmental, social, and economic variables have a crucial role. Mexican health officials recognized, on April 2021, a total of 206,146 COVID-19-related deaths.

The COVID-19 pandemic hit hard on megacities, such as the Guadalajara Metropolitan Area, a conurbation of ten municipalities with dense population settlements, significant levels of social stratification, and environmental contamination. The number of deaths is actually not as high as the media claims, but corresponds to what was expected, knowing that Mexico provides a deficient health infrastructure, limited access to social security services, and the health risk that correspond to the epidemiological profile of Mexicans. This perspective can be applied to the dynamics that the pandemic has followed and that I have witnessed in small and rural communities in Jalisco, where the population has life dynamics centered on activities of self-supply and local exchange and there is a dispersed settlement pattern that favors the low concentration of the population which has reduced infections.

In Mexico, we have survived several epidemics and pandemics, from the massive deaths in the pre-Hispanic period, due to endemic diseases such as cocoliztli or epidemic diseases such as matlazahuatl to smallpox and measles that decimated the population between the sixteenth and nineteenth centuries (Malvido and Viesca 1985, 27). On the other hand, the cholera epidemic of 1833 was very feared in Mexico by the population and the authorities; the typhus epidemic that occurred in Mexico from 1913 to 1916 ended up affecting the conception of healthcare that was held (Malvido 2003, 67).

Before the COVID-19 pandemic, another large-scale pandemic was influenza; this disease originated in a US Army camp in Kansas in March 1918 and probably in Brest, France; by August 2018, the virus underwent a genetic mutation and became a lethal virus in Mexico. During the epidemic's second wave, in October, it first attacked the populations in the north of the country and spread with great speed; the figures in a few months reached a total of sixty thousand infected. The press declared between fifteen hundred and two thousand deaths a day in Mexico in that year (Morfín and Villar 2010, 127). The Spanish influenza definitively consolidated the hygienistic discourses focused on the control, by the state, of waste and polluting emissions, as well as the strengthening of vaccination strategies, use of antibiotics, and health promotion. Some authors point out that after this drastic period for public health, the study of epidemics and pandemics adopted a biosocial approach that contributed to understanding how old diseases were replaced by new ones as a result of the inequitable conditions in which a large group remained. Conditions of insanity and misery still persist in large population groups in México (Agostini 2005).

Already in this century, during 2009 the AH1N1 flu pandemic began; Mexico was the first country to report cases of influenza A in the entire world. The pandemic spread to the United States, Canada, Spain, Germany, South Korea, and the United Kingdom (Franco-Paredes et al. 2009, 183). The germ of the virus that caused influenza (AH1N1) quickly entered the bodies of Mexicans, attacking the lung tissue and causing bleeding until death within forty-eight hours (Alonso 2010, 37). The flu pandemic caused by the influenza AH1N1 virus is presumed to have arisen in the Mexican state of Veracruz. It was popularly called swine flu, because it was considered that it had passed from a pig to a human. Today around 1,415 pathogens are known to cause disease in humans, so the relationship between ecosystem degradation and disease is not a new issue.

Gerardo Ceballos, Paul R. Ehrlichm and Rodolfo Dirzo published the article "Biological Annihilation via the Ongoing Sixth Mass Extinction Signaled by Vertebrate Population Losses and Declines," whose central argument is the loss of biodiversity due to the degradation of the structure and functions of ecosystems is directly related to the loss of human health and easily can reach the levels of pandemic and epidemics. The authors point out that we are facing the sixth mass extinction of species, which is caused by humans. The number of species that were lost in the past one hundred years should have become extinct in ten thousand years, hence the magnitude of the alarm (Ceballos, Ehrlichb, and Dirzob 2017, 6090). It is worth noting that, with regard to SARS-CoV-2, viruses are the most abundant; with high biological diversity on the planet, we still do not have enough information on their impact on public health. Morse and Schluederberg, based on their research, indicated that at least 320,000 different viruses infect mammals (Morse and Schluederberg 1990, 5).

As I have succinctly described, in the nineteenth and early twentieth centuries, there were advances in the conception of hygiene campaigns to manage and prevent outbreaks, epidemics, and pandemics. With the SARS-CoV-2 pandemic, unresolved social issues stand out in Mexico and the dimensions of environmental degradation as a driving force behind these negative events for public health. It is confirmed that inequality, overcrowding, malnutrition, environmental pollution, and poor access to social security services are elements that reduce the possibility of successfully controlling the pandemic. The current health crisis presents an opportunity for social change that favors new cultural patterns of society-environment relationship. Mexican society might reconsider new models of production, different from the extractivist production model that results on public health deterioration due to high levels of pollution and depletion of natural resocurces.

COMMUNICATION TO AVOID CONTAGION. HOW IS HEALTHCARE UNDERSTOOD IN THE CURRENT NATURE-CULTURE RELATIONSHIP?

In Mexico, the first case of COVID-19 was detected on February 27, 2020, and by April 30, 2020, there was a record of a total of 19,224 confirmed cases and 1,859 deaths, that is, a rate of mortality of 9.67 percent (Suárez et al. 2020, 466). At the national level, besides the mortality rate caused by the pandemic, deaths resulting from cardiovascular diseases, diabetes mellitus, and various types of cancer remained unchanged (National Institute of Statistics and Geography 2021, 3). Avoiding getting sick from COVID-19 as social imaginaries were instituted around the prevention of contagion above maintaining health and focused on confinement, hand hygiene, and the use of face masks. Health authorities chose to suspend face-to-face activities. Before going into confinement, I went to the office at the Regional Research Institute in Public Health and had a conversation with graduates of the nursing degree program who considered that neither Mexico nor other countries around the world were prepared to handle the pandemic and that the central thing was to educate people.

I asked the same question ofan employee of the Institute: What do you think about the coronavirus and the public health measures taken in México?

Sujeto 1. (Mujer, 55 años, viuda) ¿Tú te acuerdas de la influenza? Yo soy una persona muy espiritual, en eso creo, pienso que esta enfermedad es parte de las cosas que el ser humano genera para hacerse daño, la mente es poderosa, sobre el contagio, hay ley de atracción, si estás pensando "me voy a guardar el monedero porque me van a asaltar, ahí ya estás pensando que te van a asaltar," eso mismo pasa con el contagio en la pandemia.

Subject 1. (Female, fifty-five years old, widowed) Do you remember the flu? I am a very spiritual person, in that I believe, I think that this disease is part of the things that human beings generate to hurt themselves, the mind is powerful, about contagion, there is a law of attraction, if you are thinking "I'm going to keep the purse because they are going to assault me, there you are already thinking that they are going to assault you," the same thing happens with contagion in the pandemic.

In these first days, it was difficult for everyone to understand the controversy that started around COVID-19. As the mortality rate started to increase, there were many speculations on what were the best public health measures to overcome the pandemic. On television channels, radio, Facebook, and Twitter, there were journalists turned epidemiologists and health workers who assured that in Mexico the measures adopted by the federal government were very bad. In my opinion, I did not find negligence in the federal and state measures but at that time there was so much information circulating that it was impossible to find a clear and truthful criterion that would indicate a measured analysis.

Three months after confinement was declared, a group of students and citizens considered that the handling of the pandemic was deficient, and they expressed fear of contagion and distrust of health authorities. The main reason for confinement was, knowing the lamentable state of the health services, to avoid hospital saturation. The *Susana Distancia* communication strategy had been launched, and the goverment converted a number of facilities into special COVID hospitals to deal with severe cases of COVID-19. They also enabled institutional repositories with guidance guides and, for the first time in Mexico, since the end of February 2020, conferences were offered of daily press to report from the secretary of health the advances or setbacks in the management of the pandemic to the entire population with access to mass media of comunication. From March 16 to May 30, 2020, we remained in the first confinement, my two children attended online classes, and we established a routine with periodic activities as a mental health strategy that I accompanied with evening outings to see how how people learned about sanitary measures. Key information to prevent and avoid contagion by COVID-19 was available in public spaces through posters, to help make the disease understandable. Many shopkeepers also asked their clients to observe sanitary measures and also gave alternatives measures to contact them and to keep with their bussiness:

Later, from June to December 2020, the controversy around whether the permanent use of the mask in public spaces was a strategic input to avoid contagion displaced the fierce debates over the mortality figures for COVID-19 in Mexico and in the world. The message recovered by citizens was the mandatory use of face masks as a responsible practice of mutual care.

The federal government's health communication policy during the pandemic appealed to personal and collective awareness regarding measures to avoid contagion. President Andrés Manuel López Obrador affirmed: "forbidden to prohibit" and, despite the pressure, he did not use a mask during the informative conferences in open spaces where a healthy distance was kept, nor did he close the borders. At the local level and in some sectors of national public opinion, media employees generated a climate of horror and desolation. At the local level, the Government of Jalisco, headed by Enrique Alfaro, presumed a firm hand and faced the scandal of the murder of a young

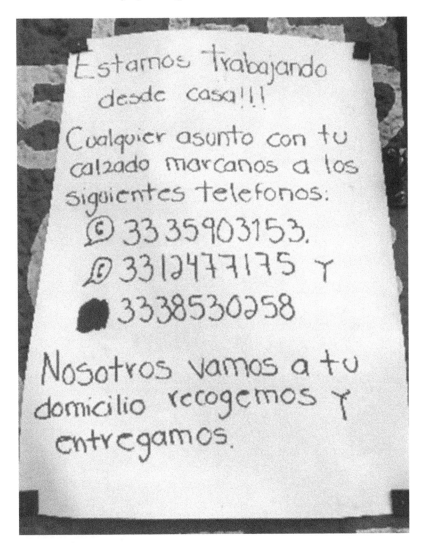

Figure 7.1. Shoemaker.
Source: Photo by the author

bricklayer at the hands of police from the metropolitan Municipality of Ixtlahuacan de los Membrillos for not wearing the mask.

As a mother, I stayed at home to care for my two children, Ezrá and Neda. They felt anxious and stressed, and we were captive spectators of the pandemic turmoil outside our home. I asked them to draw the SARS-CoV-2 virus, and both chose to draw a virus more pleasant than I imagined:

During the first two periods of confinement, in March to May 2020 and June to September 2020, my partner was working as a public official dedicated to

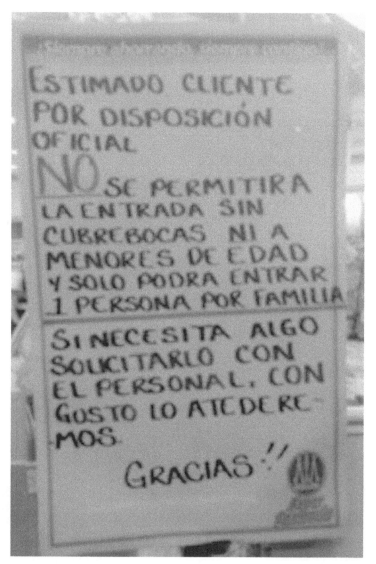

Figure 7.2.   Pharmacy.
Source: Photo by the author

operating complementary measures to maintain public health. Many people were stressed by the confinement and by the risk of contagion; one day he confided to me "in the call center they received a call from a woman who lives with her son who has Down Syndrome, she threatened to kill herself and her son, she wanted to open the gas taps. She was desperate! She accused the

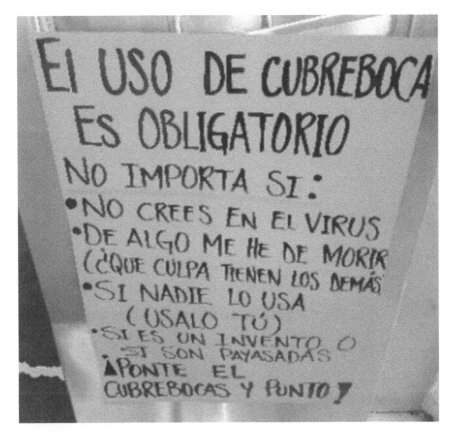

Figure 7.3. Butcher Shop.
Source: Photo by the author

neighbors, saying that no one follows the health-distance measures, she was afraid of being infected, and that she would die from COVID-19."

The continuous work in emergency situations caused breakdowns in health personnel. Everyone was afraid of being infected, despite the fact that their work did not involve contact with infected people. Government employees accused authorities of the three levels of government of not providing security equipment nor sufficient healthcare materials to carry out their work. Health workers only got a package consisting of face mask, sanitizing mats, and antibacterial gel. In an effort that implied a large national and state economic investment, a Tyvek suit was delivered to each employee to ensure better protection, a suit that they rejected exclaiming "You want us to be lynched on the street!"—this based on the fact that during the first months there were isolated attacks against health professionals. The conclusion reached in some institutional places was that only government employees with benefits and

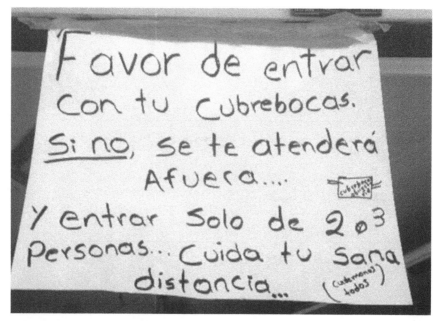

Figure 7.4.   Convenience Store.
Source: Photo by the author

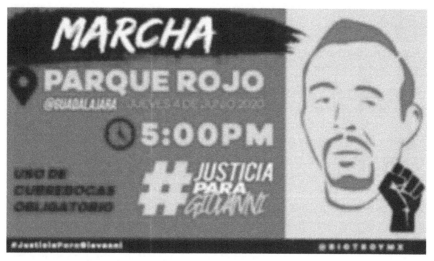

Figure 7.5.   Justice for Giovanni!
Source: Photo by the author

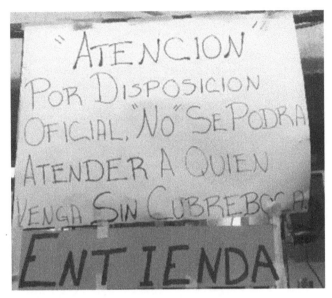

Figure 7.6. Understand!
Source: Photo by the author

contracts fell ill with COVID-19, the rest of the temporary workers, without social security, and subcontracted workers "were immune to the virus," as was also the belief of cleaning staff. As part of this popular communication to avoid contagion of COVID-19, in the third period of New Normality from October to December 2020, health professionals and other hospital employees deployed their own communication strategy to show and validate their work to prevent disease.

In other cases, humor was an alternative to cope with critical situations.

Toward the end of 2020, I had to go to the emergency department of a public hospital and I did not miss the opportunity to ask again: What do you think about the coronavirus and the public health measures that have been taken? I reproduce two answers that in my opinion were contrasting.

Sujeto 2. (Hombre de 63 años, casado) Entre otras cosas esto es parte de una conjura mundial por un conflicto entre China y Rusia, yo ya he vivido así que no me preocupa morir ¡no hay duda, es un virus que están diseminando a nivel mundial!

Subject 2. (sixty-three-year-old man, married) Among other things this is part of a worldwide conspiracy for a conflict between China and Russia, I have already lived so I do not worry about dying, there is no doubt, it is a virus that is spreading worldwide!

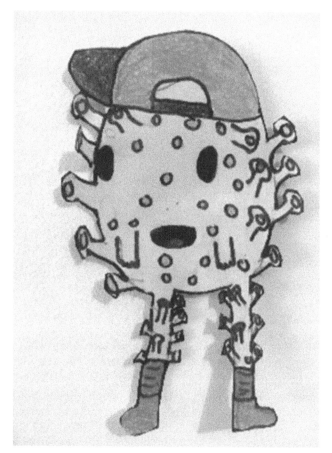

Figure 7.7. COVID-19.
Source: Author: My son, Age: 12 years, Technique: Free Drawing

Sujeto 3. (Mujer, 47 años, empleada de Gobierno, casada) Miré, como mando directivo le puedo decir que tengo dos conocidos que han enfermado de Covid 19, una es mi hermana que se contagió porque recibió a una persona que venía de España. La otra persona que contrajo el virus y se murió era el gerente de la concesionaria de BMW, tenía 57 años, la muerte ocurrió en abril de 2020.

Subject 3. (Woman, government employee, married) As a manager, I can tell you that I have two acquaintances who have fallen ill with COVID-19, one is my sister who was infected because she received a person who came from Spain. The other person who contracted the virus has already died, he was the manager of the car store BMW, he was 57 years old, the death occurred in April 2020.

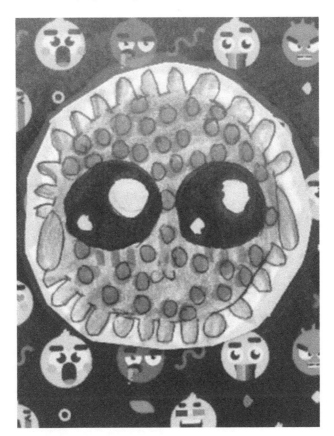

Figure 7.8. COVID-19.
Source: Author: My daughter, Age: 11 years, Technique: Free Drawing

People's opinions about how COVID-19 arose show how we imagine the virus, its contagion mechanisms, and what kind of people it "attacks." The idea of the great conspiracy that seeks to end a certain population group was surprising to me but consistent with the information memes and videos that circulated on the internet, exposing through dark humor the popular practices of healthcare, the fear of dying, and the claim of society of not having solid care institutions that guarantee the right to health and a healthy environment.

POST-PANDEMIC ADVENTURES

Tired of the confinement conditions and pressured by the commitment to deliver advances in research projects, grades, and article writing, I began to explore the possibility of resuming field work in the Agua Caliente

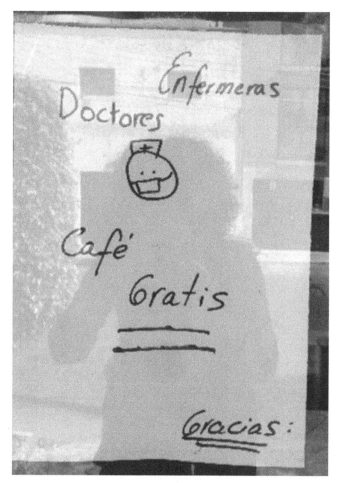

Figure 7.9.   Free Coffee.
Source: Photo by the author

community in the Poncitlán municipality in Jalisco. The first thing I did was talk by phone with the director of the Municipal Medical Services:

Yo. Buenos días Dr., ¿Cómo ha estado? ¿Cómo están las personas en las comunidades con el tema de Covid 19? ¿Muchos contagios? ¿Ya se podrá ir para allá?

Dr. S. (Médico, 50 años, casado) Buen día Dra. Estamos bien, le sugiero esperar al menos un mes más, en este momento (octubre 2020) aquí en la cabecera de Poncitlan estamos iniciando un nuevo pico de contagios y defunciones por Covid, a nivel local se tomaron medidas anticipadas, se cerró imitando al Estado, cuando no había para que, ahora las personas ya están cansadas, sus

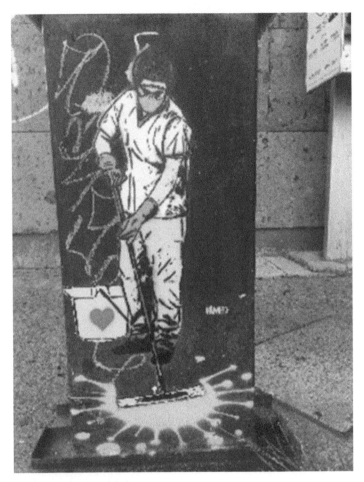

Figure 7.10.   Cleaning Employees.
Source: Photo by the author

negocios no aguantan más y están saliendo. En San Pedro Itzican si hay casos, aunque es verdad que son muy pocos y solo en adultos.

Me: Good morning Dr., how have you been? How are the people in the communities with the COVID-19 issue? Many contagions? Will you be able to go there?

Dr. S. (Doctor, fifty years old, married) Good morning Dra. We are fine, I suggest you wait at least one more month, at this moment (October 2020) here at the head of Poncitlan we are initiating a new peak of infections and deaths from COVID, locally it is They took early measures, it was closed imitating the State, when there was no reason for it, and now people are already tired, their

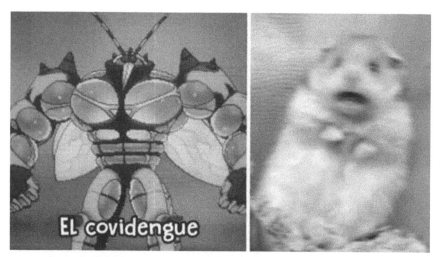

Figure 7.11. Sindemia.
Source: Photo by the author

businesses can not take it anymore and they are leaving. . . . In San Pedro Itzican there are cases, although it is true that there are very few and only in adults.

After that conversation, I decided to wait another month and on December 10, 2020, I ventured into the communities. I was surprised by what I found. In Agua Caliente, there was not one single case of COVID-19 up until January 2021, people do not use face masks, and it is impossible to adjust to some basic hygiene measures such as constant hand washing. What is kept, albeit unconsciously, is a healthy distance, given the outline of the community and the lack of spaces for community coexistence. As I was surprised by this scenario of normality, where time seemed to have stopped and COVID-19 was a ghost with which you want to scare young children, I dedicated myself to asking, so then, what has made suffer rural and marginalized families in this long period of pandemic. This is what I recovered:

The community of Agua Caliente is made up of at least 125 families who are dedicated to fishing, agriculture, and wage labor. In the community, old and new health problems coexist, and the scenario that I encountered forced me to take extreme precautions because in any case I was the vector that could introduce the COVID-19 virus into the community. Until March 2021, I had no news of cases in the community; the perception of the population of Agua Caliente around the pandemic is that COVID-19 does not exist. Older adults express their distrust toward the vaccine and toward professionals who work in municipal health institutions:

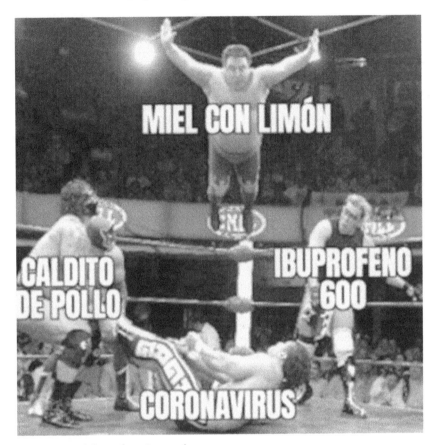

Figure 7.12.   Fight against Coronavirus.
Source: Photo by the author

Sujeto 4. (Hombre, 60 años, casado) ¿De qué nos vamos a vacunar si aquí no hay Covid? Hace unos meses mi padre ya grande de edad murió en casa dormido y cuando fui a notificar para el certificado de defunción a Poncitlán, me dijeron que iban a poner que murió de COVID 19 y ¡claro que no dije yo! Mi padre no murió de COVID ¿Con que confianza va uno a la autoridad? Mi padre no murió de eso.

Subject 4. (Male, sixty years old, married) What are we going to get vaccinated for if there isn't that? A few months ago, my old father died at home, asleep and when I went to notify Poncitlán for the death certificate, they told me that they were going to say that he died of COVID-19 and of course not! I said, my father did not die of COVID. With what confidence does go to authority? My father did not die from that.

Table 7.1.

What things have worried me during the pandemic?	
Maria is concerned that she cannot read or write.	Lidia is concerned that the children do not have classes due to the pandemic and are hanging out in the streets learning things they shouldn't be.
Juana is concerned that she will become ill with dengue or COVID-19.	
Mariana (an eight-year-old girl) worries because there is no food in her house.	Felix is concerned about pollution from burning trash and polluting the lake.
Flora is concerned about the health of her family because she has a son with asthma.	Esther worries that there is no good education, food, and security with only one patrol car.
Rosa is worried that a scorpion will bite her because there is no ambulance, and it is very difficult to leave the community when there is an emergency.	Paty is worried that there is no paid work, just a lot of unpaid work in the community.
Bertha is worried that there is drug addiction, homelessness, and alcoholism.	Ana is concerned about dengue and that there is no full-time doctor in the health center.

Note: Names are all pseudonyms.

After the confinement, some people in the community were left without work; as mobility and school attendance were restricted, families were able to count on children and young people to help in agricultural work in the land. In the words of Jonas "in 2020 the community is rich in corn and tortillas, all families got a good harvest!"

DISCUSSION

The relationship between the COVID-19 pandemic and the health of ecosystems requires specifying that viruses cause disease, but also favor biological diversity; therefore, in the case of Mexico, we must understand the havoc around the pandemic, at least around three aspects. As a first element, we must consider the continued loss of biocultural diversity and the profound inequities in the income distribution in which we live, without forgetting that where there is more environmental pollution there is also more zoonosis; second, to recognize that the epidemiological characteristics of the Mexican population follow a pattern of chronic-degenerative diseases, mental disorders, nutritional deficiencies, infectious diseases, aging, and homicides; third, the unequal distribution of health services and the lack of medical personnel.

Bruno Latour in 2020 asked: "What protection measures can we imagine so as not to return to the pre-crisis production model?" The French philosopher finds that a first measure is to give up mass consumption to become aware that the hyper-industrialized world can be suspended and the nature it is finite; the second measure is to decide to renounce production as the fundamental principle of our relationship with the world (Latour 2020, 3), a world where consumption detached itself from necessity and became a compulsion. The pandemic confirmed that in rural communities and popular areas in Mexico, old and new health problems coexist, problems attributed to environmental contamination and those products of conditions of exclusion and historical economic and social inequity. That is why Héctor Alimonda and other authors point out that we inhabit the Capitalocene, that is, we live in a geological age where war is waged on life and everything that sustains it (Alimonda, Pérez, and Martín 2017, 199).

Parents' concerns, and the concerns of rural or semi-urban families, were not focused on in international, national, and fundamentally urban discourses of the pandemic, but on the daily needs not satisfied and exacerbated by it: to continue fighting for access to first-level healthcare, maintain the right to education, guarantee respect for cultural diversity and care, access to food in sufficient and safe quantities, decent housing, and the right to decent work. Without forgetting that in a megalopolis such as Guadalajara there were numerous families who had to choose between dying of hunger or assuming a potential contagion of COVID-19.

In small communities without basic infrastructure, which have fewer than a thousand inhabitants, the pandemic arrived too late or has not arrived. What does persist and becomes worse is how girls, boys, teenagers, women, and men continue to fall ill and die from dengue, kidney disease, leukemia, and diabetes. Old diseases are not resolved while new ones are added, squeezing the space to maintain health, while the dynamics of infections seems proportional: a big city like Guadalajara is equal to millions of infections, an impoverished and marginal rural community, zero contagions. From my home, I return to the classic consideration that in Mexico there is such marginalization that these rural communities are "defended" thanks to their isolation, the distance and the deficiencies in access to social security, and of means of transportation; they become a siege that evidences an inhuman and criminal system. In July 2021, my children and husband and I fell ill with COVID-19. We first did a PCR test and then an antigen one, which confirmed the diagnoses. My children lived the experience asymptomatically, while my partner suffered from a severe fever for five days. I manifested the loss of smell and taste. We both suffered from a persistent headache, joint pain, and diarrhea. We convalesced without setbacks for fourteen days. As adults, we had been vaccinated with a single dose of the Chinese CanSino Bio vaccine in May 2021; a vaccine that the World Health Organization has not yet approved for reasons of political and economic interest, leaving public health in last place.

FINAL COMMENTS

I am far from being able to offer a discussion about the general impacts of the pandemic. However, derived from my experiences during confinement and the observation and recording work that I presented, I can affirm that the perception around the pandemic continues to build itself. For me, the balances of the pandemic in this text are the following: 1) The education of future health professionals in Mexico requires a restructuring; disease cannot continue to be understood as an exclusively biomedical problem where it is assumed that the population is ignorant on how to take care of. 2) Gender, social class, educational level, occupation, and place of residence explain the diversity of experiences and ways of caring during the pandemic. 3) Consider the impact of the communication strategy to avoid the contagion of COVID-19, in which an institutional discourse of a holistic vision where human health is equal to the health of ecosystems is absent.

We are facing a horizon to build. As Donna Haraway says, we must learn to continue with the problem (Haraway 2020, 15). The invitation is to continue with the problem in the sense of remembering and recognizing those connections and keeping up the fight to understand and avoid future pandemics. The pandemic deepened political, economic, and environmental inequalities, making them more visible, but throughout the text, in the first experiences of the pandemic, each actor poses a particular scenario to explain the emergence of the coronavirus and cope with the confinement that, paradoxically, allowed us to verify that we are all connected, humans, animals, viruses, and plants. Every actor I connected with during the pandemic, drives the need to act to transform our society-environment relationships. To avoid in the future, there are sector exclusions due to the application of political and economic criteria in personal life and public health. The pandemic showed how important it is to guarantee families an equitable distribution of wealth and offer reliable information that integrates transepistemic knowledge. The conclusion reached is in line with the holistic perspective that affirms the coexistence of communities with scientific and non-scientific knowledge. During the pandemic, the neo-extractivist market that gave certainty to society, according to the neoliberals, did not work. Profit and private enterprise do not protect people from disease and death, but rather produce and magnify them. The pandemic revealed that it is the forms of extractivist capitalism and its culture-nature relationship that stimulated the crisis, the allegory that the strongest wins showed its irrationality. As a citizen, I demand that the state recover and strengthen its leading role and that health professionals broaden their vision considering health beyond the biological field and take into account the ancestral and popular knowledge that has allowed humanity to survive.

NOTES

In Jalisco, I operate the Jalisco COVID-19 Plan as of June 2020. Once the National Day of Healthy Distance was declared concluded, we entered the New Normal regime, in that period the states were allowed, with the traffic light method, to operate measures premises for pandemic control. The Emergency Button modality did not imply a total stoppage of activities or confinements, only restriction of hours to be on the street. The first confinement by emergency button in Jalisco began in July 2020 with intermittent periods until December 2020 to receive January 2021 in confinement.

In 2009, there were no massive confinements. I was in the risk group because I was pregnant with my daughter Neda, so I spent several weeks between April and August 2009 at home, gestating and dedicated to raising my son Ezrá, who was just one year old.

I include the educational strategy of Aprende, considering that was a critical point of the contagions was the school.

Elsa Arenas. "Jalisco en aviso epidemiológico por dengue," El Occidental (Guadalajara, Jalisco) Sepetmber 20, 2019. https://www.eloccidental.com.mx/local/jalisco -en-aviso-epidemiologico-por-dengue-4208200.html

Guadalupe Martínez. "Dengue coloca a Jalisco en primer lugar a nivel nacional." udgtv (Guadalajara, Jalisco) October 3, 2019. https://archivo.udgtv.com/44lab/ dengue-coloca-jalisco-primer-lugar-nivel-nacional/ https://coronavirus.gob.mx/

REFERENCES

Agostini, Claudia. "Las delicias de la limpieza, la higiene en la ciudad de México." In *Historia de la vida cotidiana en México. Tomo IV. Bienes y Vivencias, el siglo XIX*, edited by Anne Staples and Pilar Gonzalbo Aizpuru, 563–98. Mexico City: El Colegio de México, Fondo de Cultura Económica, 2005.

Alimonda, Héctor, Catalina Toro Pérez, and Facundo Martín. *Ecologia Politica Latinoamericana. Volume II.* Buenos Aires: UAM; CLACSO, 2017.

Alonso, Carlos. "La influenza A (H1N1) y las medidas adoptadas por las autoridades sanitarias." *Desacatos no.32 Ciudad de México ene./abr* 37 (2010): 35–52.

Blanco, Mercedes. "¿Biografía o Autoetnografía?" *Desacatos, núm. 38, enero-abril* 172 (2012): 169–78.

Burns, R. Michel. "Introducción a la escritura creativa: mostrar vs. decir." In *Autoetnografía: Una metodología cualitativa*, edited by Silvia M. Bénard Calva, 197–204. San Luis Potosí: Universidad Autonoma de Aguascalientes, Colegio de San Luis, 2019.

Castoriadis, Cornelius. *Los dominios del hombre. Las encrucijadas del laberinto.* España: Gedisa editorial, 2005.

Ceballos, Gerardo, Paul R. Ehrlichb, and Rodolfo Dirzob. "Biological annihilation via the ongoing sixth mass extinction signaled by vertebrate population losses and declines." *PNAS* (2017): E6089–E6096.

Doremalen, Neeltje van, Trenton Bushmaker, and Dylan H. Morris. "Aerosol and Surface Stability of SARS-CoV-2 as Compared with SARS-CoV-1." *The New England Journal of Medicine* (2020): 1–3.

Franco-Paredes, Carlos, Carlos del Río, Peter Carrasco, and José Ignacio Santos Preciado. "Respuesta en México al actual brote de influenza A H1N1." *Salud Pública de México* 51, no. 3 (2009): 181–86.

Guarner, Jeannette. "Three Emerging Coronaviruses in Two Decades. The Story of SARS, MERS, and Now COVID-19." *American Journal of Clinical Pathology* 153, no. 4 (2020): 420–21.

Haraway, Donna J. *Seguir con el problema. Generar parentesco en el Chthuluceno.* Ciudad de México: Conssoni, 2020.

National Institute of Statistics and Geography. "Caracteristicas de las defunciones registradas en México durante enero a agostro de 2020." *Comunicado de Prensa 61/21*, January 27, 2021. https://www.inegi.org.mx/contenidos/saladeprensa/boletines/2021/EstSociodemo/DefuncionesRegistradas2020_Pnles.pdf

Koeltzsch, GK. "The Body as Site of Academic Consciousness. A Methodological Approach for Embodied (Auto) Ethnography." *Academia Letters* (2021): 1–5.

Latour, Bruno. *Trafico Visual.* June 10, 2020. https://traficovisual.com/2020/06/10/que-medidas-de-proteccion-podemos-imaginar-para-no-volver-al-modelo-de-produccion-anterior-a-la-crisis-1/.

Lim, X.Y., Y.L. Ng, J.P. Tam, and D.X. Liu. "Human Coronaviruses: A Review of Virus-Host Interactions." *Diseases* 4, no. 3 (2016): 2–28.

Malvido, Elsa. "La epidemiologia, una propuesta para explicar." *Revista de Indias* LXIII, no. 227 (2003): 65–78.

Malvido, Elsa, and Carlos Viesca. "La epidemia de cocoliztli de 1576." *Estudios Históricos, INAH* (1985): 27–33.

Morfín, Lourdes Márquez, and América Molina del Villar. "El otoño de 1918: las repercusiones de la pandemia de gripe en la ciudad de México." *Desacatos* 32 (2010): 121–44.

Morse, Stephen S., and Ann Schluederberg. "Emerging Viruses: The Evolution of Viruses and Viral Diseases." *The Journal of Infectious Diseases* 162, no. 1 (1990): 17.

Ortiz-Hernández, Luis, and Miguel A. Pérez-Sastré. "Inequidades sociales en la progresión de la COVID-19 en población mexicana." *Rev Panam Salud Publica* 44 (2020): 1–8.

Pulido, Sandra. *¿Cual es la diferencia entre brote, epidemia y pandemia?* March 12, 2020. https://gacetamedica.com/investigacion/cual-es-la-diferencia-entre-brote-epidemia-y-pandemia/.

Saltigeral-Simental, Patricia, and Ximena León-Lara. "Virus SARS-CoV-2 ¿Qué se sabe al momento?" *Acta Pediatr Mex* 41, Supl. 1 (2020): 3–7.

Suárez, V., M. Suarez Quezada, S. Oros Ruiz, and E. Ronquillo. "Epidemiología de COVID-19 en México: del 27 de febrero al 30 de abril de 2020." *Revista Clinica Española* (2020): 464–71.

Villalobos, Jenny Carolina Rodríguez. "Animales y humanos, propuesta para una sola salud." *Ciencia, Aacademia Mexicana de Ciencias* (2016): 68–75.

Villar, América Molina del. "Fuentes y abordajes metodológicos en el estudio de las epidemias: el caso mexicano." *Revista Electrónica de Fuentes y Archivos (REFA)* 9, no. 9 (2018): 78–95.

Wyatt, Jonathan, and Tony E. Adams. *On (Writing) Families. Autoethnographies of Presence and Absence, Love and Loss.* Rotterdam, The Netherlands: Sense Publishers, 2014.

Chapter Eight

Afro-Brazilians and COVID-19

Revisiting the Concepts of Necropolitics and Genocide

Siddharth Singh Monteiro Bora
and Evely Vânia Libanori

SARS-CoV-19 or COVID-19 is a zoonotic virus that causes respiratory tract infection. Beginning in 2019, the virus spread through continents within a short time, acquiring the status of a pandemic and generating one of the biggest health crises that the modern world has witnessed (World Health Organization n.d.). Within this sad and new reality, however, the victimization of socially vulnerable individuals demonstrates the incapacity of the neoliberal model in providing health and adequate living conditions and therefore life security to populations at risk.

Several studies have shown that Black individuals have been disproportionately affected by the pandemic, with higher rates of contamination, hospitalization, and mortality (Golestaneh et al. 2020). Allied to this, various research also points to a higher prevalence of chronic and neglected diseases among the Black population, which are factors associated with the worsening of COVID-19, a result of the greater social and economic vulnerability to which they are exposed (Marinho et al. 2022).

By September 3, 2022, there were 34.5 million cases with close to one million deaths in Brazil, which placed the country as one of the biggest epicenters of the disease in the world. The high incidence of contagion, added to that underreporting due to the low number of tests performed, helped the country to maintain the rate of lethality at 4.9 percent—one of the highest in the world (Brasil Ministério da Saúde 2020). The significant increase in the number of new cases of coronavirus implies the need for policies specific to minority groups living under situations of vulnerability.

Abidias do Nascimento (2019, first published in 1978) in his book *The Genocide of the Brazilian Negro: The Process of Masked Racism (O Genocidio do Negro Brasileiro: O Processo do Racismo Mascarado)* states that since its origin the formation of the Brazilian society was rooted in racial hierarchy in which the white European/Christian/white population figured on top. Considering the Afro-Brazilian reality, Abdias do Nascimento exposes the genocidal nature of the structural racism in Brazil by examining indexes of mortality, access to education and housing, and employment conditions that demonstrate the persistence of systemic racism and its impact on the demography of the Afro-Brazilian population—the idea of eliminating the Black race through a systematic strategy of destruction and subjugation.

Social segregation is a phenomenon based on racial discrimination that systematically applies action to deprive the chances of a particular racial groups to obtain "society's rewards." A racially driven system can physically, and socially, segregate individuals based on feelings of prejudice and dominance (Shihadeh and Flynn 2006). Social segregation has always been a part of the Brazilian society, and it has been a crucial factor in the reorganization of welfare and assistance in Brazil. It is often connected to low income, and it often starts from the idea of exclusion related to the territory through the connection of race and the poorest of the society. These individuals are pushed to the segregated neighborhoods and shanty towns or "comunidades" (communities) in which racial social control practices are perpetuated through "punitive sanction on blacks, brown and the poor" (Adorno 1996).

According to Mbembe (2016), contemporary forms of political and state construction are based on the need to subjugate life through the "power of death," interlocking the term "death" to the most diverse spheres of human existence. The excluded and dominated are bestowed with new and unique forms of social existence. An existence that is harsh and in inhumane living conditions that confer them the status of "living-dead," people who are deprived of social conviviality and deprive them of basic human rights (Mbembe 2016, 146). Mbembe understands that the "politics of death" are executed by the sovereign figure of the state rooted in a historical colonial logic that makes decisions about the possibility of life and death for others.

This study analyzes the overwhelming vulnerability of the Black population in Brazil during the COVID-19 pandemic. Using the theoretical arguments of Achilles Mbeme's necropolitics and Abdias Nascimento's conceptualizations on Black genocide in Brazil, I will try to demonstrate how the COVID-19 pandemic in Brazil has reinforced social paradigms of inequalities characterized by motivators of race/color and social class and perpetuated by a neocolonial structuring.

NECROPOLITICS AND DEATH
OF THE SOCIAL BODIES

Racial segregation is a systematic form of discrimination based on race which is manifest through conscious or unconscious practices that culminate in disadvantages or privileges for individuals, depending on the racial group to which they belong (Almeida 2018, 25).

In Brazil, it is possible to understand racism as an ideological weapon used for domination and exploitation of peoples (such as Blacks,[1] Indians, and others) and that has historically produced—and still produces—severe processes of exclusion and extermination of part of these populations. The racial hierarchization had a preponderant influence on the exploitation and predatory pillaging of the African continent, which also allowed the colonization and instillment of slavery in Brazil. This set of beliefs in the superiority versus inferiority of races, which is necessary to perpetuate social exclusion,[2] is still found today.

Based on the Foucauldian perspective, Mbembe (2017) conceives necropolitics as an adequate theoretical tool for understanding how to form *power diagrams*. How the processes of colonization, neocolonization, and decolonization still prevail in African, Latin American, and Caribbean contexts. According to Mbembe (2003), any historical[3] account of the rise of modern terror needs to address slavery,[4] which could be regarded as one of the first instances of a "bio political experimentation." Mbembe (2017) agrees with Foucault in conceptualizing that the mechanisms of biopower are registered in all modern states, but for him, the possibility of eliminating the *other*[5] from society is definite and present an even grimmer prospect than the one before.

According to Mbembe (2003), in such instances, power (and not necessarily state power) continuously refers and appeals to exception, emergency, and a fictionalized notion of the *Other*. In referring to it as a form of racial exclusion, he elucidates that extermination must be understood not only as the ultimate physical annihilation, but also political death, expulsion, rejection, etc.[6] It is *Death* that establishes the political space in which we live. *Death* is useful for the determination and meaning of a subjective point in the horizon of sovereignty, death ceases to be a limit to become a landmark (Mbembe 2017). The death policy operates in a systemic, objective, and timely manner, endowed with sophisticated technologies and bureaucratic actions that legitimize it.[7] The politics of death follows its own values and has *race* as its defining parameter.

Necropolitics may be understood as the various ways in which ideological weapons are deployed in the interest of the destruction through the creation of "death-worlds" that generate a new and unique forms of social existence.

These actions are legitimized under the exception of "emergencies," "problems" that justify the violation of citizens' rights and guarantees them thereby ultimately leading the opposer to their death (Mbembe 2017, 40). Under the prism of necropolitics, sovereignty becomes the struggle for autonomy and the generalized instrumentalization of human existence that is set on promoting the extinction of certain social bodies.

THE GENOCIDE OF THE AFRO-BRAZILIAN POPULATION

According to Barreto (2020), Abdias Nascimento dedicated his life to debunk the myth of racial democracy portrayed in Brazilian society. Such a myth was constructed with the help of intellectuals such as sociologist Gilberto Freyre (1946), who composed a narrative that idealized the colonization in Brazil, somewhat romanticized, that dismissed the inherent dominance, discrimination, and violence used by the settlers. The idea that slavery in Brazil was more humanitarian and benevolent, and the Blacks were seen as docile and obedient, and because of that it was possible to develop harmonious coexistence between the colonizer and the colonized, is a clear attempt to mask imperialist ideology and distort the African past, and we can also see the minimization of the oppressor's guilt and the justification of the slave system.

Nascimento demonstrates that the systemic genocide of Black populations in Brazil has been affected through mechanisms of cultural whitening that reinforce the assimilationist notion of white superiority. Therefore, the term *genocide* in Nascimento indicates a process distinct from that considered physical act.

After the end of slavery, in 1888, a large number of Black Brazilians, dispossessed and abandoned to their own fate, were seen by the Brazilian elites as a problem to be dealt with, a "black stain" (Nascimento 1978). The solution confectioned was "whitening of the Brazilian population." Such a whitening strategy touched every aspect of Brazilian society and culture, including migration, education, religion, and demographic censuses. Its ultimate goal was to limit the flourishing of Black Brazilians, and, if possible, erase their presence over the course of three or four generations (Barreto 2019).

The social model of the European colonization in Brazil saw the African descendants as problem for the evolution and improvement of the country and that therefore needed to be eradicated. The dominant sectors of the country, between the end of the nineteenth century and early twentieth century, aspired for a whiter Brazilian society, the erasure, or at least the mitigation of the "black element" in the nation's descendants.

The *Mestiços*[8] were the product of interrelation between the races. The discussion around miscegenation was of great relevance to this historic moment; miscegenation was sometimes heavily criticized and sometimes seen as a way of solution to the problem of the Black race. According to Munanga (2019) "miscegenation as solution" had the objective of creating a uniracial and unicultural society. There would be construction of a society grounded on the white racial and cultural hegemonic model, causing genocide and ethnocide of all differences, to create a new race and a new civilization.

According to Nascimento, fearing that the association of *mestiços* with Blacks would lead to making the white contingent a minority, Brazilian authorities in the beginning of the twentieth century opted for associating them with whiteness, thus hiding the significance of the African presence and influence in the country (Ramos 2019).

Against this idea, Nascimento (1978) stated that, "Despite any social status advantage such as [being an] ethnic bridge intended for the salvation of the Aryan race, the position of the mulatto is essentially equivalent to that of the black: both victims of equal contempt, identical prejudice and discrimination, surrounded by the same disdain from an institutionally white Brazilian society" (Nascimento 1978, 36). Nascimento inverted the situation by reclaiming the Blackness of those being whitewashed.

Taking that move further, he tackled another face of structural racism: cultural assimilation. He knew that whitening does not take place only through racial miscegenation or the manipulation of science and demographics. Cultural assimilation is so effective that the cultural African heritage exists in a state of permanent confrontation with the dominant system, designed precisely to deny its foundations and to destroy or degrade its structures.[9]

THE COVID-19 PANDEMIC IN THE "MODERN *FAVELAS* OF BRAZIL"

According to Pesquisa Nacional por Amostra de Domicílios Contínua data (2015), about 11.4 million people live in precarious territories, several of which are constituted by *favelas, ior comunidades*. These territories are characterized by difficulty of access, high density of buildings, and precarious and insufficient supply of essential public services, such as water and garbage collection (IBGE 2018). According to IBGE, the population residing in these territorial spaces increased by more than 60 percent between 1991 and 2010 (IBGE 2018). Considering this growth rate, it is estimated that eighteen million people currently live in favelas or other precarious territories. Other types of precarious urban housing are common in the Amazon, and in some states, there is a high proportion of these, with emphasis on *Amazonas* (35 percent), *Amapá* (22 percent), and *Pará* (20 percent) (IBGE 2020).

According to Mbembe (2003), the writing of new spatial relations (territorialization) was, ultimately, tantamount to the production of boundaries and hierarchies, zones and enclaves; the subversion of existing property arrangements; and the classification of people according to different categories, such as race. Fanon (2008) analyzes the space occupation from a colonial perspective and the division of social space into "compartments." He believes that segregation involves setting boundaries and internal frontiers, regulated by language of force, domination, and frequent and direct actions. In this sense, physical segregation,[10] as one of the elements of social segregation,[11] is essential in maintaining individuals rooted to their place of birth[12] and to certain areas of the city. According to Mbembe, "They are born there, it matters little where or how; they die there, it matters not where, nor how. It is a world without spaciousness; men live there on top of each other" (2003, 30).

In poor neighborhoods, individuals are marginalized and segregated to unhealthy spaces. Underlying the situation, Zaluar states:

Não há necessidade de fazer uma escolha racional pelo elitismo, nem de defender ideias que apoiem convenientemente a separação social entre os mais pobres e os mais ricos. Quer sequemos ou não, essa separação já está embutida nos rituais de dominação de classe e inclui um rigoroso afastamento dos locais de moradia, segregação social. (2008, 57)

There is no need to make a rational choice for elitism, nor to defend ideas that conveniently support the social separation between the poorest and the richest. Whether we dried up or not, this separation is already embedded in class domination rituals and includes a rigorous departure from dwelling places, social segregation.

In Brazil, it should also be considered that these areas concentrate populations with unfavorable health conditions, such as a high prevalence of tuberculosis, hypertension, heart disease, and diabetes in addition to the consequences of violence, expressed by high homicide rates. All these factors may exacerbate the impact of the COVID-19 pandemic in these territories. The Black population has epidemiological and social vulnerabilities that imply difficulties in accessing health services. This condition is identified in many Brazilian studies that also demonstrate difficulties in accessing health services and establish a relationship with processes of racial stigmatization. These situations generate damage to the lives of individuals, with regard to survival and health conditions.

The Brazilian Ministry of Health (2020) shows the evolution of the hospitalization rate for severe acute respiratory syndrome (SARS), analyzed according to race/color up to epidemiological week. It can be seen that the rates of SARS hospitalization among indigenous and Asian patients remained stable in all epidemiological bulletins. Among indigenous people, the lowest hospitalization rate was verified in bulletins 09 and 14 (0.2 percent) and higher in bulletin 18 (0.42 percent). Among the people of Asian race, the lowest rate was verified in bulletin 18 (1.48 percent) and the highest rate of hospitalization in bulletin 9 (2.9 percent). On the other hand, the rates of white and Black people showed significant differences.

According to the Brazilian Ministry of Health (2020), whites showed a progressive decline in SARS hospitalization rates in all newsletters of epidemiological studies, reducing from 73 percent in the epidemiological bulletin 9 to 43.3 percent in the bulletin 18. Among Black people, the hospitalization rate for SARS increased in all bulletins of epidemiological studies studied, going from 23.9 percent in the epidemiological bulletin 9 to 54.7 percent in bulletin 18.

It can be seen that the death rates from COVID-19 among indigenous and Asian patients also remained stable in all epidemiological bulletins studied. Among indigenous people, the lowest death rate was found in bulletins 14 and 15 (0.3 percent) and higher in bulletins 10, 11, 16, 17, and 18 (0.5 percent). Among people of Asian race, the lowest mortality rate was observed in bulletins 17 and 18 (1.6 percent) and the highest in bulletin 11 (2.7 percent). As with SARS hospitalization rates, COVID-19 mortality between white and Black people showed significant divergences.

People of white race/color showed a progressive decline in death rates from COVID-19 in all epidemiological bulletins published by the Ministry of Health, reducing from 62.9 percent in epidemiological bulletin 9 to 36.5 percent in epidemiological bulletin 18. Among Black people, the mortality rate from COVID-19 increased in all epidemiological bulletins studied, from 34.3 percent in epidemiological bulletin 9 to 61.3 percent in bulletin 18. Within this context, we can see that the cities most impacted by the epidemic are located in the southeast (São Paulo, Belo Horizonte), north (Manaus), and northeast (Recife, Salvador, and Fortaleza) of Brazil.

Before the end of May 2020, the governors of São Paulo and Manaus declared the eminent collapse of public health system; old social structures and deficient healthcare conditions had generated dangerous combinations. Living in segregated spaces, thousands died and had to be buried in mass graves (see Albuquerque 2020).

According to "Racial Inequality and COVID-19," by Marinho et al. (2021), in 2020 in the state of São Paulo, there was excess mortality, that is, deaths beyond expectations compared to previous years, of 127.8 percent among Blacks[13] and browns and 17.6 percent among whites. Comparatively, the most affected were young Black people up to twenty-nine years old, Black elderly people over eighty years old, and Black women (Marinho et al. 2021).

In the case of São Paulo, the most vulnerable neighborhoods have almost no census tracts and are classified as substandard or precarious habitations that are common in peripheral areas such as the neighborhoods of Capão Redondo, Pedreira, Jardim Angela, Grajau, São Rafael, Jardim Helena, Itaim Paulista, Lajeado, Cidade Tirandentes, Jaragua, and Brasilandia, among others, that characterize a situation of involuntary segregation.

A study carried out in the city of Fortaleza, located in northeast Brazil, showed that apparent lethality from COVID-19 is associated with worse socio-economic and health conditions, demonstrating the relationship between social inequalities and health outcomes in times of a pandemic (Sanhueza-Sanzana et al. 2021).

If we briefly analyze the city of Manaus, we can notice upfront that it has a high level of social segregation with low social integration. The city is composed of a high incidence of small watercourses called *igarapés*,[14] and has a lack of roads and lack of communal network, a natural and social segregated space. According to Candido et al. (2020), the lower-income classes are located near the center to the south, occupying marginal areas derived from land-filled water streams,[15] more distant areas to the north and the east, which can be noticed by the strong presence of precarious and substandard sectors in those areas.

There were 41,774 confirmed cases of COVID-19 in Amazonas through June 1, 2020; a total of 43.97 percent are from Manaus. The vast majority of these victims can identify in the cities' vulnerable communities. Adding to this delicate scenario, in Manaus, the number of deaths from respiratory syndromes and undetermined causes reached a record during the pandemic. The number of people who died by COVID-19 may be seven times greater than that officially released.[16]

According to the Manaus municipal authorities,[17] "If all deaths—from undetermined causes and syndromes—were confirmed by COVID-19, the number of deaths in Manaus could exceed 700 in the week analyzed, since the numbers of burials in private cemeteries did not enter the analysis. At least 266 deaths that occurred at home in the same period" (GLOBO 2020). Under what reasons and whose account should these deaths be linked to? The mayor of Manaus, Arthur Virgílio Neto, stated that the health network of the State of Amazonas collapsed due to the new coronavirus and that the federal government needs to expedite financial aid for those in need (UOL 2020).

CONCLUSION

In our work, we've showed that contemporary forms of political and state construction are based in "Politics of Death" that affect the most diverse spheres of human existence. Having originated from the colonial period, this morbid rationality is a racially driven *social machina* that establishes the genocidal nature of structural racism in Brazil. This idea led to a systemic and gradual process of extermination of unwanted racial groups that "tainted" the pure white/European blood. This annihilation was not perpetuated only by physical violence and rape but also through assimilation, subjugation, and religious conversion.

It is understood, then, that the historical issues and contemporary contexts produced by inequalities in different spheres—economic, social, health, transport, infrastructure, among others—have been creating an environment that puts poor populations in a more precarious situation, mainly, those who are exposed to systemic or institutional racism (Holmes et al. 2020). Differences between whites and Blacks in Brazil are easily demonstrated in data on income, education, and exposure to violence, among other indicators. Although Blacks account for 54 percent of the Brazilian population, they represent 76 percent of the poorest population (IBGE 2018).

These populations habit degenerated and disorganized spaces and are subjected to unequal distribution of catastrophes to "environmental damage." This environmental degradation tends to pass from generation to generation, an inheritance of suffering and marginalization.

The epidemiological evolution of the COVID-19 pandemic in Brazil points to a progressive increase in both mortality and hospitalizations for SARS among Black people, while revealing a sustained drop in the same rates among white people. It can thus be seen that, with the progression of the pandemic in the country, the Black population has shown itself to be in a greater situation of vulnerability.

NOTES

1. According to the IBGE, Black and brown Brazilians constitute the majority of the working class in the country. In 2018, this contingent corresponded to 57.7 million people, 25.2 percentmore than the number of white Brazilians in the workforce. In tandem, Black and brown Brazilians are substantially more represented among the unemployed and in the "informal sector," that is, those in precarious job conditions. They constitute two-thirds of all unemployed. Confirming the centrality of the racial criterion in such discrimination, the report shows that "the relative disadvantage of

this populational group remains even when one considers the cut by level of education" (IBGE 2019b).

2. The dynamics of racism in Brazil tend to be deceitful. When compared to the racial experiment in the United States, Brazil developed an assimilationist doctrine of white superiority based not on blood purity, but on phenotype (Skidmore 1992).

3. "The historical self-creation of humankind is itself a life-and-death conflict, that is, a conflict over what paths should lead to the truth of history: the overcoming of capitalism and the commodity form and the contradictions associated with both" (Mbembe 2003, 19).

4. In many respects, the very structure of the plantation system and its aftermath manifests the emblematic and paradoxical figure of the state of exception (Mbembe 2003, 21). This figure is paradoxical here for two reasons. First, in the context of the plantation, the humanity of the slave appears as the perfect figure of a shadow. Indeed, the slave condition results from a triple loss: loss of a "home," loss of rights over their body, and loss of political status. This triple loss is identical with absolute domination, natal alienation, and social death (expulsion from humanity altogether). To be sure, as a political-juridical structure, the plantation is a space where the slave belongs to a master (Mbembe 2003, 21). As an instrument of labor, the slave has a price. As a property, they have a value. Their labor is needed and used. The slave is therefore kept alive but in a state of injury, in a phantomlike world of horrors and intense cruelty and profanity. Violence, here, becomes an element in manners, like whipping or taking of the slave's life itself: an act of caprice and pure destruction aimed at instilling terror. Slave life, in many ways, is a form of *death-in-life* (Mbembe 2003).

5. According to Bauman (1998), otherness is the representation of a different group within any given company in which there is a majority. He believes that the existence of the other is fundamental to how companies establish their identity categories. He argues that identities are configured as dichotomies, such as women and men, primitive and modern, humanity and animal, man and beast.

6. "Thus, for state racism, the death of the other, the death of the bad race, the inferior race (or the degenerate, or the abnormal) is what will make life in general healthier; healthier and purer" (Foucault 1999, 305).

7. Foucault states clearly that the sovereign right to kill (*droit de glaive*) and the mechanisms of biopower are inscribed in the way all modern state's function; indeed, they can be seen as constitutive elements of state power in modernity.

8. Exploration of African women's sexuality is an important point in Nascimento theory. According to the author, the Black woman was seen as an object of pleasure by the colonizers, and currently still faces very similar problems: nowadays, the Black woman, because of her condition of poverty, lack of social status, and total helplessness, remains the easy victim, vulnerable to any sexual aggression from the white perpetrator.

9. Nascimento challenged the common notion of Catholic agency in the process of syncretism, stating that the Catholic Church was not responsible for the persistence of the African spirituality in Brazil. Its ultimate goal was to suppress the African spiritual heritage, which persisted only due to the resilience of the oppressed. That heritage persisted not only through the formation of African-derived religions but

also through other cultural expressions, such as popular religiosity and festivities. The mere incorporation of African elements by Brazilian Catholicism, though, does not deserve, according to Nascimento, to be called syncretism. It should rather be seen as a manipulative strategy of assimilation effected by "the rationalizing fertility of Brazilian racism." For Nascimento, this is nothing but the misappropriation of African culture (1978, 36).

10. The discursive construction on spatial fragmentation is an invisible mechanism of violence over specific bodies into specific locations. Social segregation, spatial segregation, economic marginalization, and mass incarceration of this group are all forms of victimization.

11. Shaw and McKay (1942) conceived the paradigm of the city as being formed from competition of social spaces and that the degeneration of neighborhoods and communal spaces and could be pinpointed through the diagrams of the level of social disorganization, heterogeneity, and social segregation in the area. Shaw and McKay (1942) understood that the ecological foundations of criminality and social disorder are laid according to the lack of macro-level social controls in a community. They understood that the crime rates were concentrated in certain areas of the city and while other regions remain relatively stable despite the continuous changes in the population and the space.

12. Colonial occupation itself was a matter of seizing, delimiting, and asserting control over a physical geographical area—of writing on the ground a new set of social and spatial relations (Mbembe 2003, 24).

13. The excess of serious and fatal cases among Blacks is explained not only by social aspects, but also by the higher prevalence of chronic diseases, such as hypertension, cardiovascular diseases, diabetes, and cancer in this population (Holmes et al. 2020).

14. An *igarapé* is a first-, second-, or third-order Amazonian watercourse, consisting of a long arm of a river or channel. There are large numbers in the Amazon Basin. They are characterized by little depth and by running almost inside the forest. Only small boats, such as canoes and small boats, can navigate the waters of a stream due to its low depth and being narrow.

15. *Riberinhos* are people derived from Black and indigenous ethnicity from the north of Brazil who live on banks rivers and are generally extremely poor and suffer from pollution from rivers and sewage. The riverside community lives in stilt houses, The activities they practice are handicrafts and agriculture.

16. According to GLOBO (2020), between April 21 and 28, the government reported that 118 deaths occurred due to the new coronavirus in Manaus, and in the same period, 262 people were buried for an undetermined cause in the public cemeteries of the capital.

17. Although the state government has prohibited the opening of trade, with the exception of essential services, the measure is not complied with. Municipal images of the East Zone of Manaus show the streets filled with people.

REFERENCES

Adorno, S. "Racismo, Criminalidade Violenta e Justiça Penal: Réus Brancos e Negros em Perspectiva Comparativa." *Racismo e Justiça penal* (1996).

Albuquerque, Ana Luiza. "Burials Triple and Manuas Cemetery Opens Mass Graves for Coronavirus Victims." *Jornal Folha de São Paulo*, April 22, 2020. https://www1.folha.uol.com.br/internacional/en/scienceandhealth/2020/04/burials-triple-and-manaus-cemetery-opens-mass-graves-for-coronavirus-victims.shtml

Almeida, S. L. *O que é racismo estrutural?* Belo Horizonte: Letramento, 2018.

Bauman, Z. *Modernity and Ambivalence*. Ithaca, NY: Cornell University Press, 1998.

Brasil Ministério da Saúde. "Painel Coronavírus." 2020. https://covid.saude.gov.br/

Brazilian Ministry of Health (Ministério da Saúde). "Indicadores de vigilância em saúde descrito segundo a variável raça/cor, Brasil." *Boletim Epidemiológico, Brasília* 48, no. 4 (2020): 1–35.

Candido, D., I. Claro, J. Jesus, W. Souza, F. Moreira, S. Dellicour, et al. "Evolution and Epidemic Spread of SARS-CoV-2 in Brazil." *Science* 369, no. 6508 (2020): 1255–60.

Fanon, F. *Black Skin, White Masks*. Translated by Richard Philcox. London: Grove Press, 2008.

Foucault, Michel Vigiar e Punir. *Nascimento da Prisão.* trad Raquel Ramalhete Ed. Petrópolis, 1999.

Freitas, V. G. *Em meio a números exponenciais da covid-19, corpos negros importam. In: Comunicação e política no contexto da pandemia: breves reflexões.* Sampaio, R. Curitiba: Compolítica / Carvalho Comunicação, 2021.

Freyre, Gilberto. *The Masters and the Slaves a Study in the Development of Brazilian Civilization.* 1st ed. NY: Zed Books, 1946.

GLOBO. "Cases of Subnotifications in Manaus" (*Com subnotificação de casos, número de mortes por Covid-19 em Manaus pode ser até 7 vezes maior*). April 30, 2020. https://g1.globo.com/am/amazonas/noticia/2020/04/30/com-subnotificacao-de-casos-em-manaus-numero-de-mortes-por-covid-19-pode-ser-ate-sete-vezes-maior.ghtml

Goes, E., D. Ramos, and A.J. Ferreira. "Desigualdades raciais em saúde e a pandemia da Covid-19." *Trabalho, Educação e Saúde, Rio de Janeiro* 18, no. 3 (2020).

Golestaneh, Ladan, Joel Neugarten, Molly Fisher, Henny H. Billett, Morayma Reyes Gil, Tanya Johns, Milagros Yunes, Michele H. Mokrzycki, Maria Coco, Keith C. Norris, Hector R. Perez, Shani Scott, Ryung S. Kim, and Eran Bellin. "The Association of Race and COVID-19 Mortality." *The Lancet* 25, no. 100455 (2020).

Holmes, Laurens, Michael Enwere, Janille Williams, Benjamin Ogundele, Prachi Chavan, Tatiana Piccoli, Chinacherem Chinaka, et al. "Black–White Risk Differentials in COVID-19 (SARS-COV2) Transmission, Mortality and Case Fatality in the United States: Translational Epidemiologic Perspective and Challenges." *International Journal of Environmental Research and Public Health* 17, no. 12 (2020): 4322.

IBGE. *Síntese de indicadores sociais: uma análise das condições de vida da população brasileira: 2019 / IBGE, Coordenação de População e Indicadores Sociais.* Rio de Janeiro: IBGE, 2019a.

IBGE. "Pesquisa Nacional por Amostra de Domicílios Contínua (PNAD Contínua 2018): rendimento de todas as fontes, 2018." 2019b. https://biblioteca.ibge.gov.br/visualizacao/livros/liv101673_informativo.pdf.

IBGE. Instituto Brasileiro de Geografia e Estatística. "Pesquisa nacional por amostra de Domicílios Contínua" PNAD-Covid 19 2020.

Lima Barreto, Maurício. "Desigualdades em Saúde: uma perspectiva global". *Ciência. Saúde colet* 22 (7) 2017.

Lima Barreto, Mauricio. "O que é urgente e necessário para subsidiar as políticas de enfrentamento da Pandemia de COVID 19 no Brasil" *Editorial Revista Brasileira de Epidemiologia* 2020 https://www.scielo.br/j/rbepid/a/6rBw5h7FvZThJDcwS9WJkfw/

Marinho, Fátima, Renato Teixeira, Hannah Arcuschin Machado, Márcia Lima, Anna Carolina Venturini, Caio Jardim Sousa, and Thayla Bicalho Bertolozzi. "Disparidades raciais no excesso de mortalidade em tempos de Covid-19 em São Paulo." Informativo Desigualdades raciais e Covid-19, 2021. https://cebrap.org.br/wp-content/uploads/2021/03/Informativo-8-Disparidades-raciais-no-excesso-de-mortalidade-em-tempos-de-Covid-19-em-Sa%CC%83o-Paulo_final.pdf.

Mbembe, A. *A Necropolitics.* Duke University Press, 2003.

Mbembe, A. "Biopoder soberania estado de exceção política da morte." *Arte & Ensaios | revista* no. 3 (2016).

Mbembe, A. *Crítica da Razão Negra.* Lisboa Antígona, 2017.

Munanga, K. *Rediscutindo a mestiçagem no Brasil: identidade nacional versus identidade negra.* Rio de Janeiro: Vozes, 2019.

Ramos, Paulo Cesar. "Nascimento, Abdias do O Genocídio do Negro Brasileiro: Processo de um Racismo Mascarado." SP Ed.|Perspectiva 2016. Revista Conexão Vol 8 # 1 (2019).

Nascimento, A. *The Genocide of the Brazilian Negro: The Process of Masked Racism (O Genocidio do Negro Brasileiro: O Processo do Racismo Mascarado).* São Paulo: Editora Perspectiva, 2019.

Sanhueza-Sanzana, Carlos, Italo Wesley Oliveira Aguiar, Rosa Lívia Freitas Almeida, Carl Kendall, Aminata Mendes, and Ligia Regina Franco Sansigolo Kerr. "Desigualdades sociais associadas com a letalidade por COVID-19 na cidade de Fortaleza, Ceará, 2020." *Epidemiol. Serv. Saúde* 2021).

Santos, Márcua Alves Dos Santos, Joilda Silva Nery, Emanuelle Freitas Goes, Aleandre Da Silva, Andreia Beatriz Silva Dos Santos, Luís Eduardo Batista, and Edna Maria de Araújo. "População negra e Covid-19: reflexões sobre racismo e saúde." *Estudos Avançados* 34, no. 99 (2020): 225–43.

Shihadeh, Edward S., and Nicole Flynn. *Segregation and Crime: The Effect of Black Social Isolation and the Rates of Black Urban Violence.* New York: Social Spectrum, 2006.

Skidmore T.E. "Fact and Myth: Discovering a Racial Problem in Brazil." Working Paper 173, April 1992, Kellogg Institute. https://kellogg.nd.edu/publications/workingpapers/WPS/173pdf.

Teixeira, Juliana Fernandes et al. "O colapso no sistema de saúde em Manaus (AM) durante a pandemia de COVID -19." *Cambiassu: Estudos em Comunicação* V.17 #30 Jul/Dez 2022. https://periodicoseletronicos.ufma.br/index.php/cambiassu/article/view/19998

Wong, Carlin, Clifford R. Shaw, and Henry D. Mackay. *The Social Disorganization Theory*. CSISS Classics, 2002.

World Health Organization. "Coronavirus disease (COVID-19) outbreak." n.d. https://www.who.int/emergencies/diseases/novel-coronavirus-2019

Zaluar, A. *A maquin e a Revolta*. Third edition. Sao Paulo: Editora brasiliense, 2008.

Chapter Nine

Language and Pandemics

Uses and Effects of WhatsApp—
Students and Teacher under Isolation

Juarez Nogueira Lins

Textual genres are constituted as instruments of social interaction—they inform, entertain, communicate ideas, and bring people and institutions together. In short, they connect everything and everyone. However, such genres are often used to disseminate lies and threats, to misinform, to discriminate, and to alienate. In this chapter, the main objective of my discussion is to analyze the uses and the effects of virtual genres particularly the use of WhatsApp by teachers and students in their daily communication under COVID-19 isolation. The data were collected from State University of Paraíba (UEPB) Brazil between October 2020 and July 2021. The theoretical foundation was based on Bakhtin (2003), Bazerman (2005), Marcuschi (2002; 2010), Coscarelli (2016), Foucault (1999), Toffler (1997), and Castells (2002; 2004). The methodological framework (based on exploratory and descriptive research) was based on Gerhardt and Silveira (2009) and Cajueiro (2013).

The research subjects were four informants, two teachers, and two students from UEPB campus in the city of Guarabira. The research platforms used for contact/data collection were WhatsApp and email. As a digital genre, the results during the pandemics were characterized by WhatsApp's diversity. As a result, among the different uses of genres there was a predominance of those that emphasized the political party differences thus "politicizing the spread" of the pandemic. The predominant subject matter emphasized was "the politization" of the pandemics accentuated by political party. The confrontation among the individuals disseminated prejudice, discrimination, and panic. Judging by the differences among them, values such as indifference

173

appeal to peaceful coexistence, laughter, anger, stress, fear, and depression were the predominant elements.

As for the procedures, through WhatsApp and email, contact and data collection (videos, audios, messages, memes, emojis, cards, stickers, etc.) were carried out. Then, these data were interpreted.

THE ADVENTURE OF LANGUAGE

Language is present in all human activities—from social-historical contexts to daily linguistic activities that characterize the most varied textual genres (Bakhtin 2003). And these genres, over time, adapt, transform, and circulate in different spheres of society. Today, in the communication and information society, or network society, new genres abound, in different virtual supports such as Facebook, Instagram, Twitter, and WhatsApp, among others (Castells 2002). These genres aim to bring people together, reduce distances, expand communication/interaction, and connect everything and everyone.

This is the main intent socially expected from the genres. However, such genres can also have unproductive uses for society. Not rarely, they often present distorted views of reality and, in this way, spread lies, threats, prejudice, and discrimination. For Marcuschi, "the impact of digital technologies on contemporary life has enormous power both to build and to devastate" (Marcuschi and Xavier 2005, 14). In this bias, the genres of the digital sphere, an unlimited source of interaction, by virtue of their reach and strength, can become "weapons" in the hands of the unscrupulous, with the purpose of manipulating, deceiving, attacking the interactants, taking them at certain times, like in the case of the pandemic, to moments of euphoria, fear, sadness, aversion, depression, etc.

In this sense, the following questions emerged guiding this research: What genres, in WhatsApp, were present in the daily lives of subjects (teachers and students) in social isolation? And how did these subjects, interacting via the social network, react to the action of these digital statements during the pandemic? In this perspective, the objective was to analyze the uses and effects of virtual genres present in the WhatsApp application on teachers and students of State University of Paraíba, Campus III, Brazil, during the period of social isolation. And so, understand how each teacher/student comes into contact with such genres.

Theoretical Framework

With the advent of the informational age (Castells 2002) and the emergence of new technologies, new digital tools emerged; social networks began to reduce distances between people, places, and access to knowledge. However, in these digital spaces, at the same time that there is a lot of information and news in real time, there are also false news and false experts in all areas; fascist, racist and homophobic postures; explicit violence; and exposure of private life. While the technological apparatus flourishes, there is a resurgence of the struggle for work, increasingly scarce, for democracy, for access to educational and cultural goods, for survival, and, above all, for power. And power, according to Foucault (1999), is action on the actions of others, to persuade even through lies as a strategy; power acts surreptitiously, today, through the networks and textual genres that inhabit this virtual space.

By discussing textual genres, Marcuschi (2010) reinforces the idea that they are diverse and adaptable to different realities and communicative situations. With the advent of the internet, new genres emerged, while others took different forms to meet the needs of the subjects in different social spheres and at different times. This assumption applies to social networks that reconfigured some genres from other media—journalistic, artistic, and other spheres—and constituted their own genres, with the purpose of promoting a change in people's daily lives (Castells 2002).

In other words, among the genres in WhatsApp groups, for example, there are those that migrated from other spheres, such as messages, and those that are in the virtual sphere, such as memes or GIFs, to mention just a few. Each one has its mark of intentionality, because human actions are not neutral. And, in the same way, "technology is not something neutral" (Castells 2002, 78). According to this finding, it is important to emphasize that each genre provides certain actions on people, leading them to develop certain actions and feelings. It is in this relationship between social networks, textual genres, and the reception of these genres that we seek to understand the effect of linguistics on social subjects in the current historical moment—the coronavirus pandemic.

Material and Method

Considering the relevance of the methodology as a way to reach a certain end (the answer to some research problem), exploratory and descriptive research was used to collect and analyze data on textual genres (digital) in the virtual environment and the action of these genres on the subjects: teachers and students of UEPB. The exploratory research aims to examine a little studied topic (text genres in the WhatsApp application, in the context of a pandemic), while the descriptive research seeks to specify important properties and characteristics of the analyzed phenomenon. As for the approach, it was qualitative and quantitative research. Quantitative because it understands the phenomenon and represents it numerically (Gerhardt and Silveira 2009).

It is qualitative because it is characterized by the qualification of the data collected during the analysis of the problem, prioritizing the perceptions of attitudes and subjective aspects of the research objects (Cajueiro 2013).

The research was carried out remotely. The research instruments used for data collection were WhatsApp and email, used to contact informants and receive the data sent (videos, messages, pictures, and memes). The research procedures were defined in five stages: first were planning, survey, reading, and systematization of theoretical data. The second was contacting the informants and collecting and systematizing data. These, sent randomly by the informants for approximately six months (November 2020 to April 2021), were cataloged by categories: videos, messages, memes, stickers, cards. The third was data analysis. What are the next two stages?

RESULTS AND DISCUSSION

A total of 241 texts (textual genres) were received from teachers and students via email and WhatsApp. Of these, teacher (A) sent seventy-nine and teacher (B) sent fifty-eight. And students (A) and (B), respectively, sent forty-eight and fifty-six. These genres were grouped and classified by categories,

Table 9.1. Distribution and Classification (Most common textual genres, in the researched groups).

Genres	Concept(s)	Q
Audio	This is a system for recording and reproducing sounds, with the purpose of communication/interaction.	14
Video	This is a recording and reproduction system of images/sounds used for interaction with the public, mainly in the digital sphere.	33
Message	Digital texts used for communication/interaction purposes and that bring together writing, images, and sounds, and can be used in email, WhatsApp, Instagram, Twitter, etc.	109
Meme	A digital genre that brings ideas, concepts, and information that spreads quickly. Through images, video, and photo words, these genres go viral in a short time.	49
Small Faces	Digital genre used to express different feelings through images created or adapted to express joy, sadness, distrust, irony, etc.	14
Charge	Journalistic/digital genre whose objective is to criticize through humor.	12
GIF	Image format that can compress several scenes and thereby display movements. Using GIFs can make emails/messages more lively, creative, and enjoyable.	10
Total		241

Source: Data collected by the researcher, November 2020 to April 2021

Table 9.2. Topics Covered by Genres

Themes	Q
Religiosity/spirituality	29
Funny situations	27
Health/diets/tips	32
Cultural	21
National and international policy	51
Tourism/gastronomy	19
Scientific	20
Family members/schoolchildren/professionals	18
Commemorative (dates/events)	06
Sexuality	14
Total	241

Source: Data collected by the researcher, November 2020 to April 2021

according to table 9.1 and also by themes (see table 9.2). The WhatsApp groups presented a diversity of textual genres typical of the digital sphere and other social spheres.

There was a predominance of messages (109), memes (forty-nine), and videos (thirty-three) in relation to other genres sent by informants (teachers and students). The messages can be classified among those of a religious nature, mostly Christian-Evangelical and Catholic; those of a political nature, left or right; those linked to humor, satirizing characters, bringing comic situations, and ironizing politics and the very condition of isolation; those linked to health issues, especially on issues related to the pandemic, such as basic care, medication tips, and expert voices; and those linked to the cultural and that point out "paths" to overcome the boredom of isolation and, therefore, bring indications of activities for confined people.

The memes sent present, in greater numbers, political/pandemic issues. In addition to the effects of a sense of humor, irony, and ridicule, memes cause controversy, because in the face of news of great impact, such as those that emerged during the pandemic, the internet bubbles with new images (Gatti 2020). As for the videos, they portray real situations—old/recent that are used and/or (re)signified, nowadays, to justify acts, build, harm images, and create new facts—and fictitious situations, with the objective of distorting facts, ridiculing people and institutions, creating false images, or provoking humor and doubts. Table 9.2 presents, more specifically, the themes explored by the virtual genres present in the WhatsApp groups.

In the information age, the technological apparatus made up of new communication tools (digital television, laptop, iPhone, smartphone), social networks (Facebook, Instagram, WhatsApp, Twitter, TikTok, and others), and the textual genres that originate and circulate from/in the virtual sphere should promote human development, but contradictorily, it also contributes to accentuating political domination and the exploitation of people (Castells 2015). And this could be evidenced, for example, in the reception of textual genres, from this digital/technological sphere, during the most critical phase of the pandemic (between 2020 and 2021).

During this period, social networks, part of this technological/informational culture, became the main instrument of interaction, bringing isolated people closer and bringing information, entertainment, and new consumption options. But not only that, the networks were also used to spread lies, fear, prejudice, intolerance, and hatred. Not necessarily because of the tension generated by the pandemic, but above all because of the climate of political polarization that has hit Brazil, since the candidacy of the former President Jair Bolsanaro and his "republic of fakes" (a common reference to the systematic use of news from social media).

In this sense, the textual genres of the virtual sphere, such as messages, videos, memes, GIFs, and others, "flooded" the homes of millions of Brazilians, bringing local, national, and global themes and concerns to the private universe of each home, or rather, the world, with its truths and lies entering through the networks and their specific textual forms, the fragile space of the subjects. These insecure and lost subjects are between political polarization, the explosion of fake news and information, and the dangers of the pandemic. Thus, understanding the use of these forms of communication/interaction (textual genres) is configured as social challenges in contemporary interactions (Rojo 2013). And in this perspective of virtual interaction, the networks made available to their users in isolation, in addition to the virtual encounter with the other, there is a wide variety of information about the social themes of that historical moment and entertainment. In the WhatsApp groups surveyed, some recurring themes were highlighted, such as national politics, health, religiosity, and humor:

- National/international policy: centered on the actions of the Brazilian former president as well as the former US president. There were fifty-one genres, including messages, videos, audios, memes, and GIFs, which addressed, in greater numbers, to the clashes between values of democracy and authoritarianism, the scientific and the religious, the "savior of the homeland" and the condemned, concern and neglect. All of them considered political insights in the face of the pandemic.
- Health: with emphasis on the pandemic moment, information on the spread of the virus, number of deaths and infections, in the world and in Brazilian regions/cities, vaccination (expectations, fear, misinformation), collective and personal care during the pandemic, symptoms, medicines, and homemade formulas.

- Religiosity/spirituality: in the face of situations of fear and impotence, people cling more fervently to their divinities, to prayers of comfort. The imminence of death, which surrounded all environments, demanded, in a way, reflections on family life, on national health, as well on human fragility in the face of natural threats and those created by humans.
- Funny situations: in an environment marked by isolation/loss of freedom to come and go, by distorted/contradictory information, fear of contagion, disbelief in institutions, doses of good humor were balms to alleviate loneliness and minimize hopelessness about the country's political destiny and the fight against COVID-19 and other viruses.

In addition to the four themes highlighted, many others were in force: cultural, family, school, and professional. These themes were, along with those already highlighted, in vogue from the end of 2020 to the end of 2021. Through the data presented, so far, it can be seen that WhatsApp groups in Brazil have become a suitable space for dissemination of political polarization, involving two national leaders, representatives of the Right and Left, respectively, former President Bolsonaro and President Lula.

Former President Bolsonaro and current President Lula were represented by deep symbols of opposition. In the end, oppositional political clashes encouraged by social media gave a fragile sense of defense and security for those who remained at home, contrary to most socially vulnerable individuals who had to expose themselves to the virus spread. These are two perspectives of interpreting the social framework suggested by the media—through education and democracy or denial. The messages exchanged among WhatsApp groups certainly strengthened the conviction that social media in times of COVID-19 "educated" the population.

Although the projects of the nations proposed by the two former presidents were entirely different, Trump and Bolsonaro were distant political bedfellows until the loss of elections of the first. Both governments were accused of destabilizing the democratic order of their nations by demonstrating strong support for authoritarian regimes, attacks on democratic institutions, and the use of fake news as strategies to remain in power. Both have in common a taste for far-right speeches and were accused of exercising open xenophobia, racism, and denial of political rights of minorities, especially women, indigenous communities, and LGBT individuals. Above all, they conducted their policies by demonstrating a severe hostility in dealing with opposing voices especially the press, dissidents, and political opponents. However, the most important feature of their government was their neglect and contempt for the human lives in dealing with the COVID-19 pandemic (Muggah 2021). As Foucault (2009, 105) emphasizes, "where there is power, there is resistance." In this particular case, the quotations can be well applied to the fierce political atmosphere during the pandemic. Still related to the Brazilian context, students sent various satirical images emphasizing the contradictory discourse of former President Jair Bolsanaro.

The cartoons were certainly linked to left-wing adversaries. Therefore, the virtual space in which these cartoons and the other genres circulated constituted symbolic spaces of a battle where the opponent groups tried to validate their perspectives. In this struggle for power, anti-ethical strategies such as the spread of fake news and misinterpretation of facts contributed to the emotional destabilization of society, in general. The increasing of tensions among antagonist groups were most of the times verbally violent and not rare disruptive among colleagues and close relatives. As a matter of power, these relations are constituted through textual genres, as well as communicative situations such as messages, memes, cartoons, videos—often with false content, half-truths, and appealing messages. And, in this way, they can cause, in subjects in isolation, different sensations (Marcuschi 2010).

Table 9.3 shows the daily common feelings in the lives of people in isolation. Stress, worry, boredom, and indifference were most emphasized followed by joy and sadness. Such data indicate that subjects in isolation were not only "bombed" by information coming from digital genres, or in a digital environment, but also experienced different sensations, from the contact with these communicative instruments.

Statements include "not leaving the house, only in case of extreme need," "It's just a gripezinha . . . (it was only a bad cold),"[1] and "There are no vacancies in hospitals for everyone." When seeing and hearing such messages, there is a certain despair, a feeling of impotence, which led people to stress, sadness, and fear. Afterwards, a message bringing a "magic formula for protection," "the Anti Covid Kit," was sold by the federal government. The scandal was rampant. The national distribution, having the president himself as "a propaganda boy," aroused the wrath of opposition leaders while renowned

Table 9.3. Teachers' and Students' Feelings in Relation to the Reception of Textual Genres in Internet Groups

Feelings	Number of Citations
Stress	4
Irritation	1
Joy	3
Sadness	2
Indifference	4
Concern	4
Depression	0
Boredom	4
Total	22

Source: Data collected by the researcher, November 2020 to April 2021

researchers went to social media to debate the inefficiency of kit. The number of deaths proved the unconcerned behavior of the president toward public health, and he also delayed vaccines acquisitions as well as providing means to public hospitals to treat the disease.

This atmosphere of doubts and misinformation got worse when the president himself defended such medication openly. It was never clear until now the relationship between the profits of pharmaceutical industry by selling such a medication and its relationship with the President, his assets or his 'parallel cabinet' financially. All that is clear is that at the crucial moments of the pandemic's spread, the president never followed the World Health Organization's direction regarding the use of mask and the importance of social distance (Ricard and Medeiros 2020).The result of this deliberate negligence and malicious intent on the part of the government in providing first the vaccine and the adoption of general guidelines to combat the disease certainly could have minimized the number of deaths in all Brazilian territories. In those moments, messages that discouraged such medications, elevated spirituality, shared pain and sadness, and increased self-esteem and value the human beings were well received.

Another option to overcome this climate of discrediting, fear, and misinformation was to send videos, memes, cartoons, and GIFs in order to minimize stress and other harmful feelings. These genres constituted two paths: laughing at the situation and making fun of it, or being indifferent. "Laughing at one's own misfortune" is something already quite common in Brazilian culture, explained by the feeling of impotence among common individuals to change the situation. Or, as the current extreme right-wing stance preaches, "God above everything and everyone," that is, in the face of situations of despair, of impotence, one seeks the divine, religiosity. The "justification," however, seems bizarre when placed in the "mouth" of the government as it seems to postpone the solution of the problem or not solving it at all by human means and therefore delivering to God's hands, the solution to exempt the ruler on duty of his inability to govern the country.

Final Considerations

The diversity of digital genres, in the virtual sphere (in the WhatsApp application), contributed to creating spaces for interaction during the pandemic. And in part, the genres—messages, memes, cartoons, videos, and others—fulfilled the objective of bringing people located in other spaces together, bringing information about political, economic, cultural, and scientific events. They managed to entertain people and feed the body and the spirit.

There was, however, the prevalence of genres that escaped, in part, the objectives of bringing people together, informing, and entertaining during the period of social isolation. In place of these human needs, many genres sought to highlight political differences—the polarization existing in the national scene between left and extreme right. Linked to this polarization were moments of irresponsibility, neglect, and chaos, represented by the image of former President Jair Bolsonaro, especially with regard to public health.

Probably as a result of this official neglect, thousands of Brazilian lives were lost. Ironically and tragically, the messianic outlook incorporated by the former president so attached to religiosity, "God above all," did not come to save its own people, but left them to their own fate. Always contrary to science, he denied the pandemic's mortal implications, spread lies, and disallowed and devalued actions to combat the pandemic. Finally, under this scenario of political and pandemic uncertainties, introduced to the population, through the media, but mainly through social networks, caused, for different subjects (teachers and students), stress, indifference, concern, boredom, and apathy.

NOTES

1. "É só uma gripezinha" (It is only a bad cold) was probably the sentence that had the most impact on Brazilians. It was uttered in a moment of commotion and stress by the president after the increasing number of deaths. The sentence not only shows the president's disregard for the pandemic but also minimized its effects, including prescribing inefficient medicine.

REFERENCES

Bakhtin, Mikhail. *Estética da criação verbal*. Fourth edition. São Paulo: Martins Fontes, 2003.

Bazerman, C. *Gêneros textuais, tipificação e Interação*. Edited by Ângela Paiva Dionísio and Judith Chamblis Hoffnagel. São Paulo: Cortez, 2005.

Cajueiro, Roberta Liana Pimentel. *Manual para elaboração de trabalhos acadêmicos*. Second edition. Petrópolis, RJ: Vozes, 2013.

Coscarelli, Carla Viana. *Tecnologias para aprender*. São Paulo: Parábola editorial, 2016.

Castells, Manuel. *A sociedade em rede*. São Paulo: Paz e Terra, 2002.

Castells, Manuel. *A Galáxia Internet: Reflexões sobre Internet, Negócios e Sociedade*. Lisboa: Fundação Calouste Gulbenkian, 2004.

Castells, Manuel. "A comunicação em rede está revitalizando a democracia." 2015. Disponível em: https://www.fronteiras.com//leia/exibir/manuel-castells-a-comunicacao-em-rede-esta-revitalizando-a-democracia. Acesso em: 19/10/2020.

Foucault, M. Vigiar e Punir: o nascimento da prisão. Twentieth edition. São Paulo: Vozes, 1999.

Foucault, M. *História da sexualidade I: A vontade de saber*. Rio de Janeiro: Graal, 2009a.

Foucault, M. "O sujeito e o poder." In *M. Foucault uma trajetória*, edited by H.E. Dreyfus and R. Rabinow. Rio de Janeiro: Forense, 2009b.

Gatti, Márcio Antonio. "Memes e o Recorte Cômico da Pandemia de COVID 19" *Revista Estudos da Linguagem* V.18, # 3 91–105. Set–Nov 2020.

Gerhardt, T.E., and D.T. Silveira. *Organizadores. Métodos de Pesquisa.* Porto Alegre: Editora UFRGS, 2009.

Marcuschi, Luiz Antônio. *Gêneros textuais emergentes no contexto da tecnologia digital.* Texto de conferência na 50ª Reunião do GEL—Grupo de Estudos Linguísticos do Estado de São Paulo. São Paulo, 2002.

Marcuschi, Luiz Antônio. "Gêneros textuais emergentes no contexto da tecnologia digital." In *Hipertextos e gêneros digitais: novas formas de construção de sentido*, edited by Luiz Antônio Marcuschi and Antônio Carlos Xavier, third edition. São Paulo: Contexto, 2010.

Marcuschi, L.A., A.M. Karwoski, B. Gaydeczka, and K.S. Brito. *Gêneros textuais: reflexões e ensino.* São Paulo: Parábola Editorial, 2011.

Marcuschi, L.A., and A.C. Xavier. *Hipertexto e gêneros digitais: novas formas de construção do sentido.* Second edition. Rio de Janeiro: Lucerna, 2005.

Minayo, M. C. de S. *Trabalho de campo, contexto de observação, interação e descoberta. In:. (Org.). Pesquisa Social: teoria, método e criatividade.* São Paulo: Petrópolis: Vozes, 2009.

Muggah, Robert. "Bolsonaro is Following Trump's Anti-Democracy Playbook." January 28, 2021. http://igarape.org.br/bolsonaro-is-following-trumps-anti -democracy-playbook/

Recuero, Raquel da Cunha. "Dinâmicas de redes sociais no Orkut e capital social." 2006. http://www.raquelrecuero.com/alaic2006.pdf

Ricard, Julie, and Juliano Medeiros. "Using Misinformation as a Political Weapon: COVID-19 and Bolsonaro in Brazil." April 17, 2020. https://misinforeview .hks.harvard.edu/article/using-misinformation-as-a-political-weapon-covid-19-and -bolsonaro-in-brazil/

Rojo, Roxane. *Escola Conectada: Multiletramentos e as TICs.* São Paulo: Parábola, 2013.

Toffler, Alvin. Távora, João (trad.). *A terceira onda.* 22. ed. Rio de Janeiro Record, 1997.

Chapter Ten

The COVID-19 Pandemic and Agency for a New Environmental Ethic

Maria Geralda de Miranda and Bruno Matos de Farias

Whatever occurs with the earth, will fall upon the children of the earth.
There's a connection in everything.

(Chief Seattle)

Elevated levels of environmental degradation and biodiversity loss have created numerous conditions for the increasing of zoonotic diseases. Many of them, such as Ebola, AIDS, and COVID-19, became viral epidemics. Most of the people affected by these viral infections are vulnerable individuals already affected by preexisting diseases (United Nations 2020, 2).

Cornanavirus belongs to a class of RNA viruses (Souza 2020, 69). These viruses attack mainly animals but also humans (Souza 2020, 69). The outbreak of the new coronavirus began in late December 2019 in Wuhan, China, with rapid spread to other continents and countries. The propensity of contamination of COVID-19, that is transmitted through air, led to isolation and quarantine measures. The World Health Organization classified the new coronavirus (Sars-CoV-2), COVID-19, a pandemic, thereby implying a disease that has spilled over across larger geographical spaces and was essentially a contagion on a global scale.

Despite all the measures, the contamination of COVID-19 in certain places of the globe such as Asia and Africa claimed the lives of more than fifteen million people worldwide and continues to disseminate itself as of this writing. Based on the premise that environmental ethics and its application are essential to the survival of the planet, the present discussion proposes first to think about the problem of COVID-19 under the light of some contemporary philosophical guidelines such as that of Peter Singer, his predecessors, and critics on the problem of the environment degradation. Second, a brief discussion will be made taking into consideration environment degradation's impact posed by the Sustainable Development Goals of the United Nations 2030 agenda.

SOME IMPORTANT ASPECTS ON PETER SINGER'S ENVIRONMENTAL ETHICS

Singer's environmental perspective proposes a "set of ethical virtues praised and the set of ethical prohibitions adopted by the ethics of specific societies will always reflect the conditions under which they (humans)[1] must exist and act, so that they can survive" (Arnold 2012, 2). Otherwise, human society would cease to exist. Singer's moral perspective goes beyond traditional thought, which includes in the context of moral action only beings considered rational and self-conscious, and who have language and thinking ability (Singer 1993, 293).

Singer widens his definition of moral action by including all animals endowed with awareness and sensitivity. In the Western cultural tradition, only people (i.e., beings endowed with indicators of humanity: self-awareness, self-control, sense of future, sense of past, ability to relate to others, concern for others, communication, and curiosity) have the right to life (Singer 1993, 294).

According to Kuhnen, Singer develops an ethics of indirect duty in relation to the environment and does so based on "the instrumental value of the environment for sentient beings and people, since he has not yet found an ethical principle consistently applicable to the environment" (Kuhnen 2004, 263).

Some non-human animals such as large primates, although not of the species *Homo sapiens*, are considered people. Singer proposes the principle of equal consideration of similar interests, a minimum principle of equality that takes into account the preferences and similar interests of beings, putting aside their physical appearance. This principle does not apply to the environment, since there is no way to identify what are the interests and preferences of non-sentient beings (Kuhnen 2004, 267).

Quoting Dworkin (1988), Kuhnen points out that the defense of the environment should be based on the idea of the intrinsic or sacred value of life, due to the historical process that gave rise to its formation (Kuhnen 2004, 268).

According to Leão and Maia, defending that only humans have intrinsic value is arbitrary. Likewise, it is not possible to deny that if there is value in conscious human experiences, one must also find value in at least some experiences of non-human beings. An object has intrinsic value if it is good or desirable by itself and not as a way of acquiring some other goal. Thus, money has an instrumental value, but our own happiness has an intrinsic value, because we desire it for itself (Leão and Maia 2010, 111). If we take as an example a problem such as the construction of a dam on a river, the decision one takes into account will be only human interests, such as the economic advantages of the dam. With a forest, we have to estimate the aesthetic or scientific value of them for humans today and in the future. If we take into account other interests besides humans, we will have to think about the animals that live in the area to be flooded, which will probably die (Leão and Maia 2010, 111).

Singer also presents some premises of defense and preservation of the environment. But the main concern will be its rare value, that is, the environment has already been destroyed by humans, therefore it became a rare instrumental entity, indispensable to the continuity of sentient beings. This justification becomes stronger when one defends a long-term environment or forest point of view. A forest takes millions of years to form and, once destroyed, its continuity is interrupted, bringing irreversible consequences for future generations.

Singer's premises in the defense of the forest concerns its economic value. The author argues that the resources that could possibly be obtained through its destruction has short-term advantages and that after a few years it will become inefficient. In many situations, economic growth must be set aside, when it implies the destruction of the environment, for its indirect consequences on the human species. Economic arguments indicate unilateral benefits of an action and are not substituted for ethical arguments (Singer 1993, 285). Still, the defense of the environment represents opportunities for recreation and "a reservoir of scientific knowledge to be acquired . . . and also because some people simply like to know that there is still a natural thing there, relatively untouched by modern civilization" (Singer 1993, 286).

Although Western civilization has difficulty in accepting long-term values, what is at stake in the case of the environment are considered "priceless and timeless values." After being lost, they cannot be recovered for any money (Singer 1993, 285). Just as the environment has a value for its rarity, it can also be valued for its beauty, because, for many people, nature provides an aesthetic sense that provides a largely inexplicable fullness. The admiration of natural beauty can cause a much greater sense of satisfaction when compared to the admiration caused by contemplation of a work of art, for example.

PETER SINGER AND BRIEF CRITICAL READINGS
RELATED TO OTHER ETHIC SYSTEMS

Singer (1993, 284) reminds us that in the Western tradition, the human species is the center of the moral universe and almost always brings together the
totality of the morally significant characteristics of this world. He quotes the
Biblical descriptions of creation in the book of Genesis to explain the higher
place occupied by human beings in the divine plan before nature. Singer sees
in the Bible itself the cultural roots of anthropocentrism, especially when
related to the idea is that man has inherited a dominion over nature and all
beings that move on earth (Viveiros et al. 2015, 333). In the book of Genesis,
chapter 26, verse 28, it is written: "God said, let us make man our image and
likeness, and let him master over the fish of the sea, the birds of the sky, the
domestic animals, all the beasts, and all the reptiles that crawl upon the earth"
(Singer 1993, 284).

The narrative described in the book of Genesis indicates that nature was
designed to serve man; this eventually generated an understanding that man
would be superior to all other creatures, and because of this he could dispose
of them as he wished them. Contrary to the Hebrew perspective, the Greeks
had moral law as an extension of nature itself. The philosopher Aristotle clari-
fies this question very well by conceiving the human beings as part of nature
and its actions linked to it. His conception of ethics is seen as an extension
of the movement of life, that is, as the vital impulse that approximates ethics
and nature (Marcondes 2009, 37).

Aristotle's ethical conception points out that the position of man in nature
is tied to the idea of *eudaimonia*. The general statement emphasized by this
concept is that the condition for the individual to have a full and complete life
depends on their constant search for their place in the universe, only then can
they acquire happiness (Aristotle 2008, 29).

In Aristotle, the concern with the insertion of man in nature is clear when
the philosopher conceives it as "endorsed with a purpose," a *"telos."* Such
a purpose is that everything that belongs to nature must realize its potency.
Aristotle's discussion on ethics for the environment is in the conception that
the human being should be seen as integrated into the environment as part of
nature, not as a separate body (Marcondes 2009, 38).

According to Marcondes, Aristotelian eudaimonica ethics influenced the
medieval model that began to order personal and social life by a set of virtues,
in search of peace and happiness with a teleological view of the world and
nature. Under the influence of Aristotelian ethics, Thomas Aquino builds a
perspective for nature by affirming that it follows a divine order. There is in
this proposition a holistic component that may be of interest to environmental

ethics. Aquinas adopts a holistic stance by stating that "knowing the order of the whole is knowing the order of the part and knowing the order of the part is knowing the order of the whole." For him, natural bodies are virtuous and any work of nature is the effect of an intellectual substance, so we see that the operations of nature are directed neatly to an end (Marcondes 2009, 38).

Descartes' "Modernity" breaks with the medieval vision of an *ordered telos* and adopts an ethics centered on the autonomy of the subject. It replaces God with man and places him at the center of the universe. In this sense, Rouanet explains, rationalism "implied faith in reason, in its ability to found a rational order, and in science, as an instance empowered to shake the game of obscurantism and transform nature to satisfy the material needs of men" (Rouanet 1993, 190).

Referring to anthropocentrism, Domanska states that it "is the attitude that presents the human species as the center of the world, enjoying its hegemony over other beings and functioning as masters of nature that exists to meet their needs." This attitude, according to the author, "is related to the type of discrimination that is practiced by man against other species" (Domanska 2013, 10).

René Descartes (1596–1650) is recognized as the founder of subjectivity and modern rationalism in which man becomes the center of the universe. This centrality of the subject, according to Mauro Grün, brought exacerbated anthropocentrism that ended up being reflected in nature in a harmful way (Grün 2009). In his work, *Descartes, Historicity and Environmental Education*, Grün analyzes the negative consequences of Cartesian philosophy for the environment. The critic considers Descartes a great villain, for being one of the responsible for the domination of nature by mechanistic science and technique. Descartes' phrase is famous, which states that with the application of his practical philosophy "we will become Lords and Possessors of nature" (Grün 2007, 36.)

Therefore, Cartesian scientific thought, based on anthropocentrism, paves the way for the development of technique and the exploration of the environment. With this, humans move further and further away from nature, subjugating it to the mere object of dominion and satisfaction of his needs as if he did not belong to it himself (Marcondes 2009).

Singer's understanding and even acceptance of a human-centered ethic can be argued in defense of the environment. To him, it presupposes an imperative to human survival. According to his understanding, there is an indirect duty to protect the environment, because its destruction has negative consequences for the human species, such as climate change and pollution and diseases.

Spinoza (2015, 155) was a staunch critic of Descartes and challenged the orthodoxies of his time with holist thought. His renewing thinking made him very close to contemporary ecological perspectives. In this way, he contributed with important presupposition to an environmental ethics that is also a moral liberation of all human tyranny towards nature. He postulated a pantheistic view of nature where everything was manifestation of a divine substace. His work *Ethics* identifies God nature; Nature and God are exactly the same.

For Spinoza, everything that exists on Earth is a manifestation of God, which he designates as Natura naturata, the ways and the manifestations of the divine essence, nature itself. The Nature of nature, that is, God, is prolonged in matter as a way of God manifests himself. "The whole nature is one individual whose parts, that is, all bodies, vary in infinite ways, without any change of the individual in its entirety" (Spinoza 2015, 155).

The philosopher traces a relationship between the Earth and the existence and suggests the necessity to restore human fidelity to the Earth and its immanence. It was the symbiosis between philosophy and holism that makes Spinoza so close to contemporary ethics and ecology. His thinking is very important and essential in the foundation of a new ethics related to the environment.

PETER SINGER'S PREMISES ON THE ENVIRONMENT AND THE UNITED NATION'S 2030 AGENDA

The international emergency, declared on January 30, 2020, by the World Health Organization has placed the COVID-19 pandemic as the worst systemic crisis ever experienced on the planet since the creation of the United Nations. As a result, the actions coordinated by governments began to focus on building fronts that considered emergency health-related challenges while combatting the deleterious effects in the health, social, and economic fields. The first UN Conference on the Environment, in Stockholm, Sweden, in 2022 became a milestone regarding international politics and a decisive step toward the emergence of environmental management policies which had an impact over countries' environmental agendas. It is written in its final report that: "Natural resources must be preserved for the benefit of present and future generations; economic and social development is indispensable to ensure man a favorable living and work environment" (CRBio07 2022).

Thus, the concept of sustainable development appears for the first time in the Brundtland Report (Instituto EcoBrasil 1987). Gro Harlen Brundtland, prime minister of Norway, was invited by the UN General Secretary and became the chair of the World Commission on Environment and Development, which was seeking a reconciliation between the environment and economic growth. Almost two decades later, after many discussions at Rio 92 and Rio+20 Global Conferences in 2015, the United Nations published the 2030 Agenda, signed by 193 countries, which reached a consensus on the Sustainable Development Goals. This agenda has seventeen Sustainable Development Goals and 169 goals, which deal not only with economic aspects of development, but also social and human. In its introduction it is written that "The Agenda 230 is an action plan for people, for the planet and for prosperity, which aims to ensure the human rights of all" (United Nations n.d.).

The Sustainable Development Goals is a broad and punctual document. By suggesting solutions to social and environmental problems we have today, it also presupposes the interdependency among nations to solve the problems that will impact the resolution of environmental problems in a positive way. The Sustainable Development Goals involve the following: 1) poverty eradication; 2) zero hunger and sustainable agriculture; 3) health and well-being; 4) quality education; 5) gender equality; 6) drinking water and sanitation; 7) affordable and clean energy; 8) decent work and economic growth; 9) industry, innovation, and infrastructure; 10) reduction of inequalities; 11) sustainable cities and communities; 12: responsible consumption and production; 13) action against global climate change; 14) life in water; 15) earth life; 16) peace, justice, and effective institutions; and 17) partnerships and means of implementation (United Nations n.d.).

The Sustainable Development Goals set universal problems and suggest some means to assist nations in achieving social security, mitigating inequalities, and ending hunger. Among the Sustainable Development Goals to be achieved is number twelve, which predicts a change in consumption and production patterns.

It is understood in a simplified way that sustainability is established as a set of human actions that aim to meet the needs of the present, without compromising future generations, based on three segments—environment, social impact, and economy—for a society or system to be sustainable. Environmental conservation, social well-being, and economic gain are also encouraged.

THE CHALLENGES TO A SUSTAINABLE ENVIRONMENT

Regarding the relationship between diseases and the environment, the document suggests that plagues are not random diseases, but a consequence of the inadequate interaction between humans and wildlife. The spread of the virus resulted in the current model that promotes the irrational use of natural resources and the *destruction of habitats*, such as forests and other areas, leading animals to change their life habits and by doing this contracting and transmitting diseases that would not exist in normal situations (Cheval et al.

2020). Situations related to environmental imbalance caused by deforestation and climate change increase the probability that zoonoses will reach levels of epidemics and pandemics (Schuchovski 2020).

According to Schuchovsky, the document points out that current political choices can outline how inequalities will be addressed. If inequalities persist and grow in shock with scenarios such as COVID-19, the aspirations of the 2030 Agenda for sustainable development can be compromised. Thus, it is necessary to restore an ethic based on respect toward the natural environment as well as the possibilities to building fairer societies. The pandemic is a real reminder of how we should think about the relationships between communities and the environment (Schuchovski 2020).

The world health crises that we are living today also implicate an environmental crisis, which in turn is triggered by the current global economic model.

Other prevalent challenges are the dominant epistemologies and hegemonic knowledge from rich countries in the north. According to Santos, they produced the Western modernity that produced a system characterized in the following way:

> As distinções invisíveis são estabelecidas por meio de linhas radicais que dividem a realidade social em dois universos distintos: o "deste lado da linha" e o "do outro lado da linha." A característica fundamental do pensamento abissal é a impossibilidade da co-presença dos dois lados da linha. O universo "deste lado da linha" só prevalece na medida em que esgota o campo da realidade relevante: para além da linha há apenas inexistência, invisibilidade e ausência não-dialética. As formas de pensamento não-ocidentais têm sido tratadas de um modo abissal pelo pensamento moderno ocidental. (Santos 2010, 48)

> Invisible distinctions are established through radical lines that divide social reality into two distinct universes: the "on this side of the line" and "on the other side of the line." The fundamental characteristic of abyssal thinking is the impossibility of co-presence on both sides of the line. The universe "on this side of the line" only prevails to the extent that it exhausts the field of reality. Beyond the line there is only no existence, invisibility and non-dialectical absence. Non-Western forms of thought have been treated in an abyssal way by modern Western thought.

Still to Santos, "a epistemologia dominante atende aos anseios das políticas colonialistas e capitalistas e entra em conflito direto com o conhecimento produzido no Sul (países da periferia do capitalismo)" ("the dominant epistemology meets the longings of colonialist and capitalist policies and directly conflicts with the knowledge produced in the South (countries on the periphery of capitalism") (Santos 2010, 48).

In this same sense, Alier previously defined nature as a kind of "hostage" to the market laws and the interests' of capital holders. Thus, the discourse of globalization is understood by him as an attempt to

> justificar ingerências ambientais dos países ricos nos países pobres ou nos países em desenvolvimento, fazendo com que o discurso de soberania tenha um viés quando imposto pelo Norte e outro quando visto pelas epistemologias do sul. (Alier 2007, 21)

> To justify environmental interferences of rich countries over the poor or developing countries North´s discourse on sovereignty is transformed and therefore is perceived differently by Southern epistemologies.

Alier-Martinez emphasizes another important point related to southern governments by suggesting that "they often do not take environmental policies seriously" thus ecologism[2] is considered "as a luxury of rich countries, before it constitutes itself as a necessity of the poor." In this sense, the author proposes the notion of "Ecologism of the Poor" that expresses not only a perspective of the environment developed according to poor countries, but also refers to the way,

> como populações discriminadas e marginalizadas (como comunidades ribeirinhas e povos indígenas e camponeses), tanto nos países ricos quanto nos países pobres, mantêm muitas vezes relações sustentáveis com a natureza. (Alier 2007, 18–19)

> how discriminated and marginalized populations (such as riverside communities and indigenous peoples and peasants), both in rich and poor countries, often maintain sustainable relations with nature.

In terms of international relations, the "Ecologism of the Poor" is based on the perception that there is an ecological debt of rich countries to poor countries. This debt arises from two distributive ecological conflicts that are different but mutually reinforcing. One of these conflicts concerns exporting from the least developed countries, acquired by the richest countries at prices that do not include compensation for externalities (Alier 2007, 287).

There is no doubt that large-scale production imposed by neoliberalism, in which unequal patterns predominate, treats nature as a mere object of consumption. Thus, one can perceive how the conceptions and needs of the capitalist system extend to the ecological field minimize the needs of Global South nations since the discourses of the dominant epistemology of the north predominate over the Sustainable Development Goals.

It is undeniable the fact that "the contemporary capitalism continues to operate for the middle of expropriation and violence, either through the expulsion of Indigenous populations from their lands or through the violence imposed in cities" (Deleuze and Guattari 1997, 10).

Ailton Krenak, one of the leading indigenous voices in Brazil, points out that:

> as práticas coloniais são poderosas porque utilizam instrumentos como a economia, que institui globalmente a posse de coisas e territórios. O autor também aponta que o pensamento indígena brasileiro traz uma crítica à modernidade e à racionalidade instrumental" (Krenack 2015, 148)

> colonial practices are powerful because they use instruments such as the economy, which globally institutes the possession of things and territories. The author also points out that Brazilian indigenous thought brings a critique of modernity and instrumental rationality[3]

Krenak also recognizes that the process of constitution of modern Western society is certainly tied to colonialism (Krenack 2015, 148).

By referring to the term coloniality of power,[4] Mingnolo states that it involves nature and natural resources in a complex system of Western cosmology in secular as well as theological terms. For this reason, "coloniality"[5] created:

> um sistema epistemológico que legitimava os seus usos da "natureza" para gerar quantidades maciças de "produtos" agrícolas, primeiro, e quantidades maciças de "recursos naturais" após a Revolução Industrial. (Krenak 2017, 8)

> an epistemological system that legitimized its uses of "nature" to generate massive amounts of agricultural "products" first, and massive amounts of "natural resources" after the Industrial Revolution.

Kopewana and Albert points out that "a compreensão do domínio da natureza, a partir da epistemologia ocidental é fundamental para deslocar e transvalorar a outra escala de saber" ("the understanding of the domain of nature from Western epistemology is fundamental to displace beyond the scale of knowledge that belongs to the Other"; Kopewana and Albert 2015, 547).

Still to Kopewana and Albert

> a compreensão do domínio da natureza, a partir da epistemologia ocidental é fundamental para deslocar e transvalorar a outra escala de saber. Uma floresta que pulsa e resplandece em suas "veias," uma humanidade ampliada pelo espectro subjetivo do perspectivismo ameríndio e por uma ecologia da natureza, dando a possibilidade de resgatar o ser humano da ignorância é levá-lo ao equilíbrio cósmico. (Kopewana and Albert 2015, 547)

the understanding of the domain of nature, based on Western epistemology, is fundamental to displace and transvalue the other scale of knowledge. A forest that pulsates and shines in its "veins," a humanity amplified by the subjective spectrum of Amerindian perspectivism and by an ecology of nature, giving the possibility of rescuing human beings from ignorance is to leading them to cosmic balance.

Developing Kopewana and Albert's perspective, Viveiros de Castro states that

> Essa transvaloração pode ser pensada a partir do perspectivismo amerídio, que busca a ecologia da natureza em oposição à ecologia humana ocidental que se assenhora da natureza. A ecologia da natureza amerídia busca reintegrar o ser humano a condição de pertencimento a humanidade ampliada entre seres viventes e não-viventes. (Viveiros de Castro 2014, 140)

> The valorization of nature can be understood by taking into consideration Native American perspective that considers the ecology of nature opposed to Western ecology. Therefore, Native American ecology seeks to reintegrate the human being into the condition of belonging to humanity expanded between living and non-living beings.

Probably having in mind the Amerindian and other non-Western systems, Estermann suggests also that: "é necessário caminhar no sentido oposto, de percebermos outras formas de, reordenação da lógica para outra ética de valores, para vislumbrar outro estado de coisas" ("it is necessary to walk in the opposite direction, to perceive other forms of understanding, by reordering the logic thought to another kind of ethics and values to envision another state of things"; Estermann 2006, 109).

Viveiros de Castro emphasizes the differences between Western philosophy and Native American cosmology when confronted, leading us to conclude that: "os humanos são animais que ganharam alguma coisa, já para os ameríndios, os animais são humanos que perderam alguma coisa"/ "humans are animals that have gained something, but for Native Americans, animals are humans who have lost something." Still, to Viveiros de Castro, Western thought lost the capacity to see the humanity of other beings as well as to integrate the intuitive spirits of forests and rivers. In other words, humans deny the world of life and its differences.

Summing up, Castro understands Native American cosmology as a project of planetary development and sustainability. This ancestor project has much to teach since its foundations are based on the premise that all beings of nature are sacred. According to her perspective, there is an interaction between all beings since all of them interconnect with the cosmos (Viveiros de Castro 2008, 95).

To Viveiros de Castro, Native American epistemology is relevant to the planetary integrity regarding the sustainability of the planet. Today, the context experienced by Western societies demonstrate that their social-political and economic projects make it impossible to humans to harmonize with nature. Thus, the search for planetary sustainability implies in understanding the socio-environmental web.

The cultural approach of Edward Said on multiculturalism criticized the integration of all society into hegemonic cultures without modifying the structural matrix of society that seeks to relativize the other, and produces a model of development and sustainability based on a culture of consumption and objectification of nature. To him, although multiculturalism proclaims respect for diversity, its bases are still based on models that presuppose the inferiority of the culture of the other, that is, to treat as irrelevant what is different from the Western model (Said 1996, 56).

According to Kopewana and Albert, the logic of multiculturalism must be reversed, and one way out is to break the excessive needs of the market and neoliberal policies, because they still orbit within this model of negative sustainability based on the predation of nature (Kopewana and Albert 2015, 547).

The current production model has established a pattern of human development that can be called poor development, because it favors a minimal portion of the world's population, which is, as Peter Singer would say, "a lack of ethics" since only a small portion of people enjoy the planet's natural resources. In the document entitled *Human Rights, Environment and COVID-19* of the UN Environment Programme, it is clear that:

> a crise da covid-19 revela uma verdade clara sobre riscos catastróficos em um mundo cada vez mais globalizado: uma resposta efetiva requer ação preventiva imediata, ambiciosa e baseada em evidências em nível internacional. (United Nations 2020, 5)

> the crisis of COVID-19 reveals a clear truth about catastrophic risks in an increasingly globalized world: an effective response requires immediate, ambitious and evidence-based preventive action at the international level.

With a view to preventing possible future global threats, like the pandemics, the right to a balanced and sustainable environment on which we all depend for our health and well-being is a fundamental human right. And the United Nations warn that

> a abordagem sobre os direitos humanos é necessária para abordar os impactos desiguais da crise da Covid '9 sobre as pessoas pobres, vulneráveis e

marginalizadas, além de outros fatores subjacentes, incluindo a degradação, a mbiental. (United Nations n.d.)

The human rights-based approach is needed to address the unequal impacts of COVID-19 crisis on poor, vulnerable and marginalized people, as well as other underlying factors, including environmental degradation.

As Leão argues, economics and ethics are relevant areas today, one of which is the rights of the environment, since it is a problem that concerns our daily life, and that has gained importance in the last fifty years. For Singer, to the extent that someone lives according to ethical standards, it should justify them not only in terms of personal interest, but in terms of that acts based on personal interest are compatible with ethical principles pertaining to a larger audience (Leão and Maia 2010, 17).

An Aristotelian vison of the environment would presuppose "technical or instrumental knowledge," through which the human being interferes in the environment, must be subordinated to rational, *prudential decision*. One can observe the contemporaneity of the Aristotelian thought, if we consider Singer's critique on the fundamentals objectives of the United States in the face of a degraded environment, the loss of planetary biodiversity, hunger, and diseases (such as zoonosis); the United Nations, as an international political body that is, through guidelines to countries and people, seeks to prevent the conditions of human life on the planet from becoming more difficult or even unfeasible. The preservation of the environment today is related to an intergenerational issue; it is about enabling future generations to know something untouched by human action. Singer reflects on the ethical responsibility of this generation to future generations, which justifies a long-term action. One should therefore choose a course of action that has the best consequences for all those affected, after examining all possible alternatives. This utilitarian attitude is an initial basis on which we come to universalize decision-making based on ethical interest.

CONCLUSION

The pandemic caused by COVID-19 is an alert for global societies to consider the patterns of consumption and exploitation in relation to the natural environment. Epidemics prior to COVID-19, such as Ebola, avian flu, swine flu, zika, and others virus manifestations, demonstrate how the planet can face soon other global pandemics. According to Singer (1993), it is necessary to discuss ethical issues, taking into consideration Native American thought and cosmology in which all beings are sacred and interrelate. This is the basic step to think about a sustainable planet. According to Native American perspective, there is no place for destruction of biomes, because countless beings would lose (as they have already lost) their homes. The same ethics of sacredness is applied to the rivers and oceans of the planet, places of life and not of death by unnatural extinction caused by human action. Anthropocentric perspective is leading the planet to exhaustion because of the predatory ways that the current production model was imposed. The premises contained in the United Nations' 2030 Agenda point out concerns with ethnic minorities and motivations of gender equality, preservation of the environment, and the reduction of social inequalities. It includes prerogatives toward hunger, diseases, and unemployment, especially related to countries in the Global South. However, the document does not question the predatory economic model that implement the destruction of biomes and its transformation into products that will be sold on stock exchanges like commodities. This model perpetuates Global South continuous roles as providers of material resources to northern countries. The wealth generated by such exports only benefits few countries but the environmental damage is shared by all.

Matida argues that after several global forums (Rio+20, Eco92, among many others), it is urgent to design and implement public policies that, through a broad process of capacity building, "translate the commitments expressed in the statements to face inequities in health, from actions on the social determinants of diseases" (Matida 2016, 1940). Matida is right. If we do not question the foundations of the current model, based on other ethical thoughts, such as the Native American, for example, public policies will not reach the causes, but only the consequences. The health crisis is at the same time, as mentioned earlier, a mirror of the environmental crisis, which in turn is a reflection of the current global economic model, which brought the world to this historic moment in which the COVID-19 pandemic claimed thousands of lives around the world.

In this way, it is important to emphasize that we will not be able to end and/or avoid new pandemics if we do not adopt actions that will imply decision-making with regard to nature conservation and harmonious coexistence with it. It is necessary to think and transform man-nature relations. This transformation requires new epistemologies and political imagination beyond the intellectual and political exhaustion of the north.

NOTES

1. Our emphasis.

2. Martínez Alier demonstrates how, in practice, the uses of the terms ecologism and environmentalism vary: "in Colombia, environmentalism is more radical than ecologism; in Chile or Spain, the opposite happens" (Alier 2007, 21).

3. According to Pereira (2021, 148), Krenak starred in one of the historical moments of the struggle of the original peoples when he spoke during the Constituent Assembly in 1987. He painted his face black in protest against the setbacks of indigenous rights and the omission of the Brazilian government that used/uses the justification of economic advancement to continue denying and silencing the original peoples, making indigenous peoples a target throughout the country.

4. The coloniality of power is a concept interrelating the practices and legacies of European colonialism in social orders and forms of knowledge, advanced in postcolonial studies, decoloniality, and Latin American studies, most prominently by Anibal Quijano.

REFERENCES

Allier, Joan Martinez. *O Ecologismo dos Pobre: conflitos ambientais e linguagem de valoração.* São Paulo: Contexto, 2007.

Arnold, Luiza. "Desenvolvimento Sustentável: direito fundamental ao ser humano." 2012. https://egov.ufsc.br/portal/conteudo/desenvolvimento-sustent%C3%A1vel -direito-fundamental-ao-ser-humano

Aristotle. *Ética a Nicomaco.* Brasília: UnB, 2008.

Cheval, Sorin, Cristian Mihai Adamescu, Teodoro Georgiadis, Mathew Herrnegger, Adrian Piticar, and David R. Legates. "Observed and Potential Impacts of the Covid-19 Pandemic on the Environment." *International Journal of Environmental Research and Public Health* 17, no. 11 (2020): 4140.

CRBio-07. "Uma Só Terra: Conferência de Estocolmo completa 50 anos." June 5, 2022. https://crbio07.gov.br/noticias/uma-so-terra-conferencia-de-estocolmo -completa-50-anos/

Descartes, René. *Discurso do Método.* Translated by João Gama. Lisboa: Edições, 2007.

Deleuze, Gilles, and Félix Guatari. *Mil platôs: capitalismo e esquizofrenia.* São Paulo: Editora 34, 1997.

Domanska, Ewa. "Para Além do Antrocopentrismo nos Estudos Históricos." *Revista Expedições:Teoria da História e Historiografia* V.4, N.1, Jan––ulho 2013.

Dworkin, Ronald. *El domínio de la vida.* Barcelona: Ariel, 1998.

Estermann, Josef. *Filosofía andina: sabiduría indígena para un mundo nuevo.* 2 ed. La Paz: ISEAT, 2006.

Grün, Mauro. *Ética e Educação Ambiental: a conexão necessária.* 11 ed. São Paulo: Papirus Editora, 2007.

Grün, Mauro. "Descartes, Historicidade e Educação Ambiental." In *Pensar o Ambiente: bases filosóficas para a educação ambiental,* edited by I. C. M. de Carvalho, M. Grun, and R. Trajber. Brasília: Ministério da Educação, Secretaria de Educação Continuada, Alfabetização e Diversidade, UNESCO, 2009.

Kopenawa, Davi, and Albert, Bruce. *A queda do céu: palavras de um xamã yano-mami.* São Paulo: Cia das Letras, 2015.

Krenack, Ailton. *A vida não é útil.* São Paulo: Cia das Letras, 2015.

Kuhnen, Tânia Ap. "Do valor intrínseco e de sua aplicabilidade ao meio ambiente." *ethic@,* Florianópolis 3, no. 3 (2004): 255–73.

Instituto EcoBrasil. "Nosso Futuro em Comum - Relatório Brundtland." 1987. http: //www.ecobrasil.eco.br/site_content/30-categoria-conceitos/1003-nosso-futuro -comum-relatorio-brundtland

Leão, Igor Zanoni Constant Carneiro, and Denise Maria Maia. "O valor do meio ambiente segundo Peter Singer." *Capa* 6, no. 4 (2010).

Machado, Cristiani Vieira, Adelyne Maria Mendes Pereira, and Carlos Machado de Freitas. "As respostas dos países à pandemia em perspectiva comparada: semel-hanças, diferenças, condicionantes e lições." *Políticas E Sistemas De Saúde em tempos de pandemia: nove países, muitas lições.* Rio de Janeiro, RJ: Observatório Covid-19 Fiocruz; Editora Fiocruz, 2022, 323–42.

Marcondes, Danilo. "Aristóteles: ética, ser humano e natureza." In *Pensar o Ambiente: bases filosóficas para a educação ambiental,* edited by I. C. M. de Carvalho, M. Grun, and R. Trajber. Brasília: Ministério da Educação, Secretaria de Educação Continuada, Alfabetização e Diversidade, UNESCO, 2009.

Matida, Álvaro Hideyoshi. "Por uma agenda global pós-Objetivos de Desenvolvimento do Milênio." *Revista Ciênc. Saúde Coletiva. Rio de Janeiro* 21, no. 06 (2016): 1939–46.

Pereira, M. S. et al. "Da criação aos tempos da pandemia da Covid-19." *Revista Docência do Ensino Superior* (Núcleo Docente Estruturante da Enfermagem da UFMG) Belo Horizonte, v. 10, p. 1–19, 2021.

Rouanet, Sergio Paulo. *Mal-estar na modernidade.* São Paulo: Companhia das Letras, 1993.

Said, Edward W. *Orientalismo: o Oriente como invenção do Ocidente.* Tradução de Tomás Rosa Bueno. São Paulo: Companhia das Letras, 1996

Santos, B. S. "Para além do pensamento abissal: das linhas globais a uma ecologia de saberes." *Revista crítica de ciências sociais,* n. 78, 2007.

Seattle Chefe. "Preservação do meio ambiente - manifesto do Chefe Seattle ao presi-dente dos EUA." Translated by Magda Guimarães Khouri Costa. São Paulo, Babel Cultural, 1987.

Singer, Peter. *Ética prática.* São Paulo: Martins Fontes, 1993.

Souza, Ligia da Paz de. "A pandemia da COVID-19 e os reflexos na relação meio ambiente e sociedade." *Revista Brasileira de Meio Ambiente* 8, no. 4 (2020): 68–73.

Spinoza, Baruch de. *Ética.* Translated by Grupo de Estudos Espinosanos; edited by Marilena Chauí. São Paulo: Editora da Universidade de São Paulo, 2015.

Schuchovski, M. "Covid-19 e o Novo 'Normal.'" 2020. http://www.madeira-total.com.br/artigo-da-dr-a-em-ciencias-florestais-mariana-schuchovski-covid -19- e-o-novo-normal/

United Nations. *Indicators of Sustainable Development: Guidelines and Methodologies.* Third edition. New York: United Nations, 2007.

United Nations. "E-government Survey: Digital Government in the Decade of Action for Sustainable Development with Dddendum on COVID-19 Response." 2020. https://digitallibrary.un.org/record/3884686

United Nations. "About Our Work to Achieve the Sustainable Development Goals in Brazil." n.d. https://brasil.un.org/pt-br/sdgs

United Nations. Millennium Development Goals Report for Solomon Islands, 2010c https://www.undp.org/pacific/publications/millennium-development-goals-report-solomon-islands-2010

United Nations. "Direitos Humanos, meio ambiente e Covid 19. Programa para o meio ambiente." n.d. https://www.ohchr.org/sites/default/files/COVID19_PO.pdf

Viveiros, Edna Parizzi, Maria Geralda de Miranda, Ana Maria Pires Novaes, and Kátia Eliane Santos Avelar. "Por uma nova ética ambiental." *Eng. Sanit. Ambient.* 20, no. 3 (2015): 331–36.

Viveiros de Castro, Eduardo. *Cannibal Metaphysics: For a Post-structural Anthropology.* 1 ed. Minneapolis: Univocal Publishing, 2014.

_____. "Perspectivismo e multinaturalismo na América indígena". *O que nos faz pensar Rio de Janeiro*, v. 14, n. 18, 225–254, 2018.

Chapter Eleven

Biopolitics and Environmental Governance in the Time of the New Coronavirus Pandemic

Marcus Alexandre Cavalcanti and Kátia Eilane Santos Avelar

On March 11, 2020, the World Health Organization (WHO) declared a pandemic state due to the disease caused by the SARS-CoV-2 virus, which was named COVID-19.[1] The first months of 2020 were marked by the rapid increase in the number of infected people worldwide. The pandemic has had direct effects on the control and management of populations, such as measures to contain the spread of the disease, effectiveness and support capacity of health systems, and socio-economic measures to serve the most vulnerable populations (Cavalcanti et al. 2020). Although the pandemic has caused serious inconvenience to the planetary community,[2] there were some positive aspects of the quarantine that have brought benefits to the environment. Scientists around the world have been realizing that the drop in movement in big cities has brought some beneficial aspects, such as the reduction of pollutant emissions in large cities, the fall in the production of commercial waste, and reduction of pollution in the oceans. These and other consequences of the reduction of human circulation and its impact on the environment have been reported and are important factors for reflections on the planet's environmental issues.

In this way, this chapter seeks to verify how the social isolation measures recommended by the WHO, due to the new coronavirus pandemic, have impacted the environment. We assume that the measures adopted have been positively affecting the environment. The question that guides this chapter is the following: What positive impacts has social isolation brought to the environment?

To adequately answer this question, we will analyze the complexity of the pandemic in its multiple dimensions, considering climatic, socio-economic, political, scientific, and cultural factors that shape the entire scenario of the pandemic. Such analysis will be conducted from authors such as Edgar Morin, Michel Foucault, Felix Guattari, and Enrique Leff. The work has a qualitative approach and involves a bibliographic survey, as well as documentary instruments.

In the first part of the chapter, we will present Foucault's notions of government and biopolitics to deal with the management of public policies aimed at caring for populations during the COVID-19 pandemic and in Enrique Leff and his proposal for an environmental rationality. Such a proposal makes it possible to think about the right to life, to culture, to environmental protection so that new ways of being in and with nature can be built. Next, we will rely on the complex thinking of Edgar Morin and the notion of ecosophy of Feliz Guattari, both French thinkers who propose a sustainable planetary project. In the third section, we intend, through bibliographic studies and documentary records, to point out the main positive aspects that the social isolation imposed in the pandemic has brought to the environment.

GOVERNANCE IN THE PANDEMIC TIME

The declaration of the pandemic caused by the new coronavirus, COVID-19, on March 11, 2020, generated worldwide repercussions by exposing planetary vulnerability in relation to population health, as well as correlated government practices. The expression "novel coronavirus" refers to severe acute respiratory syndrome coronavirus-2 (SARS-CoV-2) and is explained by the fact that there are hundreds of viruses belonging to the coronavirus family. As this new virus was first identified in December 2019, in the city of Wuhan, China, it came to be called coronavirus disease 2019, or COVID-19 (Lone and Ahmad 2020).

Some hypotheses have been raised in order to understand how the emergence of COVID-19 occurred. Many researchers maintain that it arose due to human interference in nature, mainly by the removal of wild animals from their natural habitat for commercial purposes. Others claim that globalization, with the consequent expansion of urban centers, degradation of the natural environment, and destruction of habitats, was the reason for the emergence of the pandemic (Oliveira et al. 2020; Nascimento et al. 2020).

For Chaves and Bellei (2020), measures are needed to prevent the occurrence of future new outbreaks and to maintain an ecologically balanced environment, with preservation of environmental reserves. The fact is that, for the authors, the predatory intervention of humans in the environment is among the main causes of the occurrence of the pandemic. The confrontation of the current pandemic is compromised by the widespread impacts of social distancing, quarantine, and lockdown measures, which affect the physical, mental, social, and economic dimensions of the population, plus the uncertainties of the evolution of the epidemic itself and the responses of individuals, communities, and leaders' policies.

Thus, it is possible to see that from the beginning, COVID-19 emerged as a biopolitical problem that required direct action by the state and its agents to contain it. The WHO has defined the new coronavirus as a pandemic of global proportions and considers that fighting the pandemic will be ineffective if it does not take into account the multidimensionality of the problem and if it does not involve the full participation of all local and global people.

Actions such as closing borders, travel restrictions, distancing, and social isolation have shown good results in combatting the spread of the virus (Oliveira et al. 2020; Nicola et al. 2020; Ramonet 2020).

The pandemic began to highlight the importance of managing public policies aimed at caring for the populations, while it pointed out the need for changes in the forms of government in the midst of the crisis. The notion of government[3] that we refer to in this text is in line with the Foucauldian perspective that understands it as the art of exercising government, of directing the conduct of individuals through practices of normalization and control of their actions. The government, according to the author,

is constituted by the institutions, procedures, analyses, reflections, calculations and tactics that allow the exercise of a specific and complex form of power that has the population as its main target, as a way of knowing the political economy and as an essential technical instrument security device. (Foucault, 2008, 143)

Government actions are reticularly distributed across the social fabric and are evident in the various measures imposed by the government, such as the suspension of various activities, the reduction in the movement of people and means of transport, as well as the retraction of consumption habits that are reflected in the economy, society, and environment. Government takes place around political actions aimed at encouraging and improving the population's living conditions.

Such measures are configured as biopolitical actions, since they use strategies that affect the population to stimulate and increase the lives of individuals. Biopolitics would be a form of population governance aimed at predicting state actions based on the evaluation of statistical data related to their vital behaviors—mortality, birth rates, rates of contamination by infectious

diseases, vaccination campaigns, hygiene models, sanitation, control of epidemics, level of health, duration of life—such processes are assumed through
a whole series of interventions and regulatory controls, etc. The population
becomes the object of biopolitics (Foucault 1988).

Biopolitics is a technology that emerged between the end of the eighteenth
century and the beginning of the nineteenth century, which is part of liberal
political rationality. This new technology became a fundamental category for
the analysis of society (Foucault 1998). Foucault (1998) points out that

> Biopolitics focused on the species body, on the body permeated by the mechan-
> ics of the living being and as a support for biological processes: proliferation,
> births and mortality, the level of health, the duration of life, longevity, with
> all conditions that can make them vary; such processes are assumed through a
> whole series of interventions and regulatory controls: a biopolitics of the popu-
> lation. (Foucault 1988, 152)

Based on forecasts, estimates, statistics, and measurements, it will prioritize
interventions in phenomena at a global level, with the intention of establishing regulatory mechanisms. These issues, therefore, become essential
elements for state interventions, especially the norms that will guide society. Investment in the life of the population becomes a way of increasing
and enriching the strength of the state itself (Foucault 1988). According to
the author,

> It also seeks to verify the resources of the environment (nature, climate, soil
> salubrity, water purity), while supporting not only the quality of life but also
> the maintenance of humanity itself. We then realize that biopolitics is based on
> practices that are aimed at the control of groups of individuals, that is, the popu-
> lation becomes the central axis for the effectiveness of government. In this way,
> any action on the part of the State affects the populations. (Foucault 1988, 140)

Foucault (1988) conceives that biopolitical governance takes place from a
rationality that affects the life of populations and cities. By rationality, the
author understands the sets of calculated prescriptions that organize institutions, produce knowledge, distribute spaces, and regulate behaviors; in this
sense, rationalities induce a series of effects on the real.

Inspired by Foucault, Leff (2010) elaborated a rationality directed to environmental issues. This rationality presupposes a reform of the entire existing social structure, be it political, state, productive, or legal (Leff 2010).
Environmental rationality in Leff

> involves an environmental theory to explain reality through a resignification of
> concepts, techniques and instruments aimed at sustainability. Finally, it involves

a method of urban management materialized in self-management, a radicalism that combines empowerment, politicization and social participation of social strata jettisoned by the market. (2002, 282)

The process in which we are immersed is dominated by a formal and instrumental rationality suited to the capitalist mode of production. According to Leff, environmental rationality is opposed to this model, constituting itself through the articulation of four modes of rationality, namely substantive, theoretical, technical, and cultural. Environmental rationality is an alternative to the contemporary hegemonic process. Substantive rationality would be "The axiological system of values that regulate actions and guide social processes for the construction of an environmental rationality based on the principles of ecologically sustainable, socially equitable, culturally diverse and politically democratic development" (Leff 2002, 130).

Theoretical rationality "builds the concepts that articulate the values of substantive rationality with the material processes that support a productive rationality based on ecotechnological productivity and an environmental potential for development" (Leff 2002, 130).

Technical rationality is that "which produces the functional and operational links between the social objectives and the material bases of sustainable development through an adequate technological system, legal procedures for the defense of environmental rights and ideological and political means that legitimize the transition to environmental rationality, including the power strategies of the environmental movement" (Leff 2002, 130).

The fourth mode, according to Leff (2002), is cultural rationality:

A system of meanings that produce the identity and internal integrity of the different cultural formations, which give coherence to their social and productive practices; these establish the singularity of heterogeneous environmental rationalities that do not submit to a general environmental logic and that demand meaning and reality at the level of local actions. (Leff 2002, 130)

These four articulated levels of rationality constitute the basis of environmental rationality. In this way, the construction of environmental rationality would be a process that involves different instances of thought. The core of this proposal requires, above all, a change in the way of looking at environmental issues and finding ways to solve the problems related to this area. Among the various issues that are correlated with environmental rationality are the constitutions of capitalist societies, which, in his opinion, are not prepared to deal with environmental complexity, insofar as the vast majority of legal dictates were created to benefit companies and the exploration of nature, and not themes that demand social and environmental projects. This new rationality, supported by greater autonomy and individual and cultural freedom in the face of bureaucratic policy formulation, could break the traits of mere environmental management posed by the colonial perspective of international environmental policies (Leff 2002). For Leff, it is necessary to go beyond legal reforms and the expansion of rights; that is, it is necessary to create new laws that consolidate the right to life, to culture, to environmental protection so that new ways of being can be built in and with the nature. The author also emphasizes the need to restore the relationship between society and the environment to promote favorable conditions for human survival, based on sustainable development[4] premised on the revaluation of economic, ethical, and aesthetic relationships in the environment around human beings and the values of democracy, justice, and human coexistence before nature.

COMPLEXITY, ENVIRONMENT, AND ECOSOPHY

Complex thinking arises with the challenge of instituting another way of seeing the world and nature, by overcoming modern (Cartesian and simplistic) thinking. According to Morin (2013), we need to restore the disjunction between society and nature, a result of modern Western thinking. According to Morin (2013), the solutions to respond to socio-environmental problems are not just technical; they need our way of thinking to reform to encompass the society/nature relationship in its complexity and engender the changes demanded by our society. It is thought of as a broad and diffuse network that involves a multiplicity of interconnected nodes; the complex thought of French sociologist Edgar Morin also brings a reticular conception. Complexity[5] (woven together) proposes that reality should be treated as a dynamic network of interactions that consider the multiple determinations of the real. Morin (2000), when dealing with complex thinking,[6] states that society and nature form an inseparable whole. In the words of the French thinker,

> There is complexity when different elements are inseparable constitutive of the whole (such as the economic, the political, the sociological, the psychological, the affective, the mythological) and there is an interactive and inter-retroactive interdependent fabric between the object of knowledge and its context, the parts and the whole, the whole and the parts, the parts themselves. Therefore, complexity is the union between unity and multiplicity. (Morin 2000, 38)

It is a thought that integrates the environment, society, culture, and economy with the political, which considers the complexity of interrelationships as well as the hologrammatic character, that is, that the whole is in the parts and each part is in the planetary whole (Morin 2008). The complexity of the environmental issue requires a broad methodological approach that overcomes the limits of systematized knowledge determined by the discipline of the various areas of knowledge that compartmentalize knowledge (Morin 2008).

Morin (2008) advocates that the problems of the planetary age are transversal, multidimensional, transnational, and global, and are demanding a reform of thought and teaching that makes it possible to face them. This is because the fragmentation of reality prevents us from seeing the global and the essential, and also makes it difficult to understand the problems in a context that is planetary. The challenge of the planetary community is the creation of a conscience that can face all forms of predation and destruction to the environment by the capitalist model and that makes possible a model of sustainable life. For this, it is necessary to create measures that make it possible to reduce the production of solid waste; that combat the degradation of rivers, oceans, and other water sources; and that contain the increase in atmospheric pollution, deforestation, and fires that contribute to global warming and climate change. In this sense, the pandemic of the new coronavirus presented itself as a kind of brake on the contemporary exploratory and predatory model.

Thus, Morin (2008) highlights the relationships between phenomena that involve the field of environmentalism, but also the socio-cultural and economic field, both necessary for the preservation of society and the planet.

When citing the connections and relationships that lead us to think about the pandemic and its consequences for the environment, we also highlight the proposal of the ecologist Félix Guattari, who states that the environment must be thought of transversally through the articulation of what he classifies as Three Ecologies. Its perspective consists of the articulation between the three ecological registers (that of human subjectivity, that of social relations, and that of the environment) to clarify the environmental problem (Guattari 2009). Guattari (2009) also explains that,

> The link between social, mental and individual ecology is not intended to encompass all these heterogeneous ecological approaches in the same totalizing or totalitarian ideology, but to point out the opposite, the perspective of an ethical-political choice of diversity, of creative dissent, of responsibility towards of difference and otherness. (Guattari 2009, 31)

The articulation of these three ecologies is what the French ecologist calls ecosophy. Guattari's (2009) ecosophical thinking makes it possible to minimize the risks of environmental problems and human interventions in nature. Ecosophical thinking enables reflection and understanding of the development of new social practices, making man a being capable of interacting with the environment. This reflection subsidizes the deepening of ethical norms and social premises of human action in the environment. Ecosophy is the study of the relationship between nature and human beings, proposing discussions between the environment, man, and social relationships. It is a search for concrete actions, taking into account man's interaction with the environment. Ecosophical thinking consists of awakening the individual to the serious ecological imbalances of contemporaneity (Guattari 2009).

Thus, the conditions of the environment cannot be dissociated from our condition of existence on the planet. This condition is directly associated with our ecological formation, our formation as an environmentally conscious subject. For Guattari (2009), the human being needs to learn to develop a transversal thinking to understand the fragile relationships that govern the global aspects of our planet, in a broader sphere and the local and pertinent aspects to our development. Very close to this conception, we find the thoughts of Leff (2002), who proposes the notion of ecological globalization that is driving the creation of new social organizations to face this existing ecological degradation, and at the same time, this new form of social organization questions the legitimacy of the state and its actions in relation to socio-environmental issues. This movement demonstrates the crisis of the state in the face of issues such as justice, equity, democracy, and the environment (Leff 2006).

THE POSITIVE IMPACTS OF THE CORONAVIRUS PANDEMIC ON THE ENVIRONMENT

Since the COVID-19 pandemic began, many isolation actions to prevent the spread of the virus have been employed. Such measures have had positive impacts on the environment. Biopolitical governance practices have gained centrality in the ongoing pandemic. Individuals and populations had their daily lives altered by practices that were previously unthinkable in the current social order. There was a reasonable deceleration of the productive forces, adoption of practices of isolation, and social distancing. A series of government actions were taken in order to provide protection to the lives of the population and individuals. The rulers were asked to position themselves in economic, social, political, sanitary terms, and their positions had planetary repercussions. Rescuing Foucault's analyses, we can see that in the pandemic, the relationship between individuals and the environment constituted a crucial point of biopolitics.

To a large extent, this position was taken in the fight against COVID-19. And, in this sense, much of the governmental attention was spent on intervening in ways of acting collectively in the face of such risk. The biopolitics-oriented approach had as main protagonists the health, science, and education sectors that advocated unconditional care with the preservation of life. As argued so far, the role of state government in the life of populations and cities in the context of COVID-19 is remarkable.

The restrictions triggered by social isolation have also demonstrated some positive impacts for the environment around the world. Braga et al. (2020) point out that the limit on car circulation in large cities caused a drastic decrease in the release of pollutants, such as carbon dioxide and nitrogen dioxide, thus improving air quality in several parts of the world. significantly. According to the National Aeronautics and Space Administration and the European Space Agency, air pollution in some countries, such as the United States, China, Spain, and Italy, among others, was reduced by up to 30 percent during the lockdown periods (Muhammad, Long, and Salman 2020).

Satellite images have shown that the coronavirus pandemic is lowering air pollution levels around the world. The European Space Agency has also detected a reduction in nitrogen dioxide, a chemical compound that contributes to air pollution and acid rain. Nitrogen dioxide is a result of emissions from cars and other industrial processes and can, among other things, cause respiratory problems (Universidade Federal de Juiz de Fora 2020).

The impacts suffered by air transport agencies were also very visible; this was due to the guidelines given to the population to stay at home and remain in isolation. They caused the biggest crisis the international airline industry has ever faced. Demands around flights dropped dramatically during the pandemic (Rodrigues 2020). In the first three months of 2020, there was a decrease of sixty-seven million passengers in Europe compared to the previous year. In the United States, domestic air traffic dropped by about 40 percent. While cancellations were more frequent around the world than in the United States, states have not instituted restrictions on domestic air travel. In Brazil, for both domestic and international flights, the drop was much more significant, reaching approximately 92.5 percent in the number of passengers transported on domestic flights and 97.3 percent on international flights (Furlanis, Santos, and Araujo 2020).

It is important to emphasize that, according to the European Environment Agency, the plane is considered the most polluting means of transport in the world and represents 3.5 percent of the impact caused by global warming. Each aircraft emits 258 grams of carbon dioxide per passenger with the burning of kerosene, in addition to the set of other gases and negative effects that contribute to global warming. The authors found that greenhouse gas emissions also declined in the pandemic. Here, we highlight the need to practice new forms of biopolitical governance that imply the valorization of life, the preservation of the environment, the strengthening of social solidarity, the practice of public policies, and the adoption of new cultural habits which favor a more harmonious relationship between human beings and the environment.

For water resources, positive effects were detected, such as the improvement in water quality in different parts of the world, some of them publicized by the media, as was the case observed in the waters of the Venice canals in Italy between the months of July 2019 and December 2020. Residents celebrated this event on social media, including reporting the appearance of fish. In an interview with the American channel CNN, the city hall said that this happened due to the decrease in the movement of boats. In India, studies were also carried out to assess the effects of the lockdown on air and water quality. The studies were carried out in city of Ghaziabad, considered the second largest industrial hub in Uttar Pradesh. Scientists observed that restrictions due to transport activities, as well as industrial ones, brought a significant decrease in the concentration of atmospheric pollutants, reaching an 85 percent reduction in the concentration of particulate matter 2.5 in the city, which is considered one of the most polluted cities from across India (Lokhandwala and Gautam 2020). Scientists also found that with restrictions to contain the spread of the novel coronavirus, the waters of the River Ganga were considered fit for drinking. This improvement in quality is mainly related to the closure of industries and the consequent interruption of the release of their waste directly into the river. After this considerable improvement, fish and other species of marine life could once again be seen in its waters (News18 2020).

In this way, it was possible to verify that social isolation generated a series of developments that positively impacted the air and water, and that such changes directly affected issues related to health, hygiene, and biodiversity, thus reaching all the inhabitants of the planetary community. Morin (2000) believes that these movements establish new arrangements for the emergence of an ecological ethics, whose developments make it possible to become aware of local and global responsibilities, having as a central point the respect for life and the defense of the right to it in a world without geopolitical boundaries. In this movement, the feeling of belonging to humanity and to a single planet is amplified.

In Brazil, the effects of reduced human activities, as well as social isolation, on air quality were also observed in several capitals. Pereira, Silva, and Solé (2020) carried out surveys in the main Brazilian cities and concluded that the effects of the isolation caused by the pandemic led to a large decrease in pollution levels. The authors point out that in the period of partial stoppage in the cities of São Paulo and Rio de Janeiro, between the months of January and July 2020, the air quality in the urban areas decreased drastically in the concentrations of carbon dioxide when compared with the monthly average of the last five years. Atmospheric pollution rates in the city of São Paulo were reduced by around 50 percent in just one week, thus reducing the number of people with respiratory syndromes. Such facts cast a glance at the complexity and at the ecosophical perspective, since the reduction of human exposure to environmental pollution consequently led to a decrease in related respiratory problems. The pandemic highlighted the relationships that health has with the environment and social planning, a moment for the design of new biopolitical strategies of governance with care for life. Foucault (2008), when referring to control strategies, emphasizes their importance around this new reality.

Changes were also observed in the fauna of large centers as a result of the reduction in human circulation during the pandemic. Places that were once dominated by human presence began to be visited by wild animals such as pumas, coyotes, and turkeys in the United States; wild boar in Spain; leopards in several places in India; and deer in Japan, all examples of recent sightings recorded in the urban areas. After nearly ten years of unsuccessful mating attempts, Hong Kong's empty zoo has recorded this act occurring naturally between a pair of pandas, something that could be advantageous for the conservation of this species. In Italy, sheep and wild boar were photographed walking peacefully through empty streets. In Japan, a group of deer was seen roaming the streets in the city called Nara. *The Guardian* newspaper (2020) published that "it is not uncommon for people to see the increase in the presence of insects and animals, even in urban areas." The fact is that, with isolation to prevent the spread of the virus, wild animals began to occupy urban spaces.

Guattari (2009) states that the solution to avoid the occurrence of future problems related to pandemics is the maintenance of an ecologically balanced environment, with the preservation of environmental reserves. For him, one of the consequences of the degradation of the environment is the emergence of wild animals in urban spaces, since the environment is extremely sensitive to human activities.

A survey carried out by the Brazilian Institute of Geography and Statistics in 2020 pointed out that 91 percent of the Brazilian industry had negative impacts on their sales due to the COVID-19 pandemic. Data show that 76 percent of industrial companies have reduced or paralyzed production. The sectors that described the greatest decrease in demand were clothing (82 percent), footwear (79 percent), furniture (76 percent), construction (73.1 percent), and services (71.9 percent), especially services provided to families (84.5 percent). Retail had a drop of 70.8 percent in sales, with emphasis on the sale of vehicles and motorcycles. Entrepreneurs identified that there was a 77 percent decrease in the supply of raw materials and inputs for production, mainly because of the transport system, which made access to inputs or raw materials necessary for production difficult (Brazilian Institute of Geography and Statistics 2020).

Morin (2003) draws attention to the financial uncertainties that the world has been facing due to the emergence of the coronavirus. The author takes the opportunity to point out the uncertainties generated by the pandemic, not only economic, but in relation to the future of the planet. He thus proposes the creation of new ways of relating to the environment. Leff points to the need for an environmental rationality "that signals the possibility of restoring the organicity between nature and society, transcending the predominance of the instrumental use of reason when understanding the environment as complexity" (2001, 136).

Another important factor of extreme importance that contributed to the reduction of environmental degradation was the drop in the movement of people in the cities. This phenomenon was reflected in the production and recycling of waste. In the city of São Paulo, for example, during social isolation, there was a 56 percent drop in waste collected by sweeping the streets and a 12 percent reduction in the collection of common household garbage. Selective collection also increased by 25 percent. This number shows that people started to adhere more to recycling and the correct destination of garbage during the pandemic period. These positive environmental effects are, once again, proof that the responsibility to preserve the environment is in the hands of each individual (CG Ambiental n.d.). Here emerges as the main factor the awareness and participation of subjects in the processes of environmental transformation, performing acts of care and preservation that will improve the quality of life of all living beings, an environmental rationality, based on a new ethics, with principles based on a democratic life, values and cultural sociocultural actions that are capable of mobilizing and reorganizing society as a whole, "in a process of reappropriation of nature, orienting its values and potentials towards a sustainable and democratic development" (Leff 2004, 143).

For this rationality to be really built, it is necessary to develop complex thinking, through the articulation of different fields of knowledge, disregarding the fragmentation of reality that resist and prevent such a path of completeness (Morin 2016). It is about putting into practice actions that are forged by ecosophical thinking, that consider the multiple determinations for a sustainable future, an environmental knowledge that goes beyond existing conditions and transforms knowledge for the construction of a new social order. It is about proposing a biopolitics that considers life, not only from the point of view of the present, but also full of practices aimed at the best future of the planet.

CONCLUSION

In view of the discussion in this chapter, we can see that there have been considerable positive changes in relation to the environment caused by the pandemic. The restrictive measures recommended by the WHO, due to the new coronavirus pandemic, allowed greater attention to issues related to the environment, thus promoting reflections on the gradual process of environmental deterioration.

Through this process, awareness can be awakened for the invention of behaviors that allow sustainable coexistence throughout the planetary community. The survival of all depends on the development of a socio-environmental perspective that considers Guattari's ecosophical proposal, which advocates the awareness that everyone must care for and preserve the environment for future generations. These values, coupled with environmental rationality, can provide benefits in relation to the quality of life and reveal planetary complexity, providing transversality—that is, the interactions between the environment, culture, politics, economy, health, and education—for the taking of actions that positively affect the environment.

NOTES

1. Coronaviruses (CoV) are a large viral family, known since the mid-1960s, that causes respiratory infections in humans and animals. Generally, coronavirus infections cause mild to moderate respiratory illness, similar to a common cold. Most people become infected with the common coronaviruses throughout their lives. All coronaviruses are transmitted from person to person, including SARS-CoV, but without sustained transmission. Some coronaviruses can cause severe respiratory syndromes, such as severe acute respiratory syndrome (SARS). SARS is caused by the SARS-associated coronavirus (SARS-CoV),

2. The concept of planetary community, coined by Morin (2018), considers humanity as a family that engages in the search for social equality for all and acts responsibly in relation to the environment because it feels integrated with the Earth.

3. By forging the notion of governmentality, Foucault (1995) proposes a terminology to designate and analyze the activity that consists of governing the conduct of men in a context and through state instruments without having to resort to any concept of state or the notion of government institution.

4. In a simplified way, sustainable development can be defined as human actions that aim to meet the needs of the present, without compromising future generations. In addition, it is based on three elements: environment, social impact, and economy. Therefore, it is understood that for a society or system to be sustainable, environmental conservation, social well-being, and economic gain must be encouraged.

5. The word complex is taken from the Latin complexus and complecti which mean "what is woven together" (complexus) or "what contains different elements" (complecti).

6. Complex thinking proposes three principles to overcome current thinking. The first of these is the recursive principle, in which product and effect are necessary for production and causation. Thus, any process whose final states or effects produce the

initial states or initial cause. The second is the dialogical principle, which links antagonistic and contradictory terms to know reality, and the third is the hologrammatic or holonomic principle, which states that there is no only the part is in the whole, but the whole is also in the part (Morin 2005, 108).

REFERENCES

Agência Européia de Meio Ambiente. "Redução da poluição no ar durante pandemia convida à mudança de comportamento social." n.d. https://ec.europa.eu/jrc/en/research-topic/environmental-monitoring

Braga, F., G. M. Scarpa, V. E. Brando, G. Manfè, and L. Zaggia. "COVID-19 Lockdown Measures Reveal Human Impact on Water Transparency in the Venice Lagoon." *Science of the Total Environment* 736 (2020): 139612.

CG Ambiental. "Pandemia do Coronavírus: 3 impactos ambientais positivos." n.d. https://www.cgambiental.com.br/blog/pandemia-do-coronavirus-3-impactos-ambientais-positivos

Cavalcanti, Marcus Alexandre, Eliane Cristina Tenório Cavalcanti, Elisabeth Da Silva Almenara, and Nathan da Costa Cavalcanti. "A Pandemia do novo coronavírus (Covid-19): Considerações sobre o neoliberalismo e o Estado de Bem-Estar Social nas ações governamentais." *Rev. Augustus. Rio de Janeiro* 25, no. 52 (2020): 94–111.

Chaves, T.do S.S., and Bellei, N.C.J. "SARS-COV-2 O Novo Coronavirus: uma reflexão sobre a sáude única e a importância da medicina de viagem na emergência de novos patógenos." *Revista de Medicina* 99, 1 (fev) 2020.

Foucault, M. *Dits et écrits*. Paris: Gallimard, 1995.

Foucault, M. *História da Sexualidade, vol. 1 A vontade de saber*. Nineteenth edition. Rio de Janeiro: Editora Graal, 1988.

Foucault, M. *O Nascimento da Biopolítica*. São Paulo: Martins Fontes, 2008.

Furlanis, A. M., D. N. Santos, and M. N. Araujo. "Covid-19 e os impactos no fluxo de passageiros no Brasil: O caso do aeroporto internacional de São Paulo." In: *FatecLog, 2020, Bragança Paulista*. Congresso Internacional de Logística, 2020.

Gattari, F. *As três Ecologias*. 20 ed. Trad Maria Cristina F. Bittencourt. Papirus: Campinas, 2009

Guattari, Félix. *Qué es la Ecosofía?: textos presentados y agenciados por Stéphane Nadaud*. Buenos Aires: Cactus, 2015.

Leff, Enrique. *Epistemologia Ambiental*. 3 ed. Cortez São Paulo, 2002

Leff, Enrique. *Saber Ambiental:sustentabilidade, racionalidade, complexidade, poder* 3. ed. Vozes: Petrópolis, 2004.

Leff, Enrique. *Racionalidade ambiental: a reapropriação social pela natureza*. Rio de Janeiro: Civilização Brasileira, 2006.

Leff, Enrique. "Complexidade, racionalidade ambiental e diálogo de saberes." *Educação & Realidade, Porto Alegre* 34, no. 3 (2009): 17–24.

Leff, Enrique. *A Complexidade Ambiental*. 2 ed. Cortez São Paulo, 2010.

Leff, Enrique. *Saber ambiental: sustentabilidade, racionalidade, complexidade, poder*. São Paulo: Editora Vozes, 2014.

Lone, Shabir Ahmad, and Aijaz Ahmad. "Covid-19 Pandemic: An African Perspective." *Emerg Microbes Infect* 9, no. 1 (2020):1300–08.

Lúcia, M. E. *Orth*. Petrópolis: Vozes, 2001.

Lúcia, M. E. *Racionalidade ambiental: a reapropriação social da natureza*. Translated by Luís Carlos Cabral. Rio de Janeiro: Civilização Brasileira, 2006.

Lokhandwala, Snehal, and Pratibha Gautam. "Indirect Impact of COVID-19 on Environment: A Brief Study in Indian Context." *Environmental Research* 188 (2020): 109807.

Morin, Edgar. *Os Sete Saberes Necessários à educação do futuro*. 8 ed. Cortez São Paulo, 2000.

Morin, Edgar. *Terra-Pátria/ Edgar Morin e Anne-Brigitte Kern*. Translated to French by Paulo Azevedo Neves da Silva. Porto Alegre: Sulina, 2003.

Morin, Edgar. *Introdução ao Pensamento Complexo*. Instituto Piaget Lisboa, 2005.

Morin, Edgar. *Ciência com Consciência*. 11. Ed. Rio de Janeiro: Bertand Brasil, 2008.

Morin, Edgar. *A Via para o Futuro da Humanidade*. Rio de Janeiro: Bertrand Brasil, 2013.

Morin, Edgar. *Introdução ao Pensamento Complexo*. Translated by Ilana Heineberg. Porto Alegre: Sulina, 2016.

Morin, Edgar. *A cabeça bem-feita: repensar a reforma, reformar o pensamento*. Translated by Eloá Jacobina. Rio de Janeiro: Bertrand, 2018.

Muhammad, Sulaman, Xingle Long, and Muhammad Salman. "COVID-19 Pandemic and Environmental Pollution: A Blessing in Disguise?" *Science of the Total Environment* 728 (2020): 138820.

Nascimento, Vagner Ferreira do et al. "Impacto da COVID-19 sobre o trabalho da enfermagem brasileira: aspectos epidemiológicos." *Foco* (Brasília) 11(1 n.esp): 24-31, ago. 2020.

News18. "Ganga River Water Has Now Become Fit for Drinking as Industries Remain Shut Due to Lockdown." April 20, 2020. https://www.news18.com/news/buzz/ganga-river-water-has-now-become-fit-for-drinking-asindustries-remain-shut-due-to-lockdown-2575507.html.

Nicola, Maria, Zaid Alsafi, Catrin Sohrabi, Ahmed Kerwan, Ahmed Al-Jabir, Christos Iosifidis, Maliha Agha, and Riaz Agha. "The Socio-economic Implications of the Coronavirus Pandemic (COVID-19): A Review." *International Journal of Surgery* 78 (2020): 185–93.

Oliveira, Marcel Nunes, Maria Amávia de Souza Campos, and Thomaz Décio Abdalla Siqueira. "Coronavírus: globalização e seus reflexos no meio ambiente." *BIUS-Boletim Informativo Unimotrisaúde em Sociogerontologia* 20, no. 14 (2020): 1–12.

Pereira, M. U., C. A. M. Silva, and D. Solé. "COVID-19 and Air Pollution: A Dangerous Association?" *Allergologia et Immunopathologia* 48, no. 5 (2020): 496–99.

Ramonet, I. "Ante lo desconocido. La Pandemia y el sistema-mundo." *Le Monde Diplomatique Edición Chilena*, 30 de abril de 2020.

Rodrigues, L. A. "Transporte Aéreo de Passageiros e o Avanço da Covid-19 no Brasil." *Revista Brasileira de Geografia Médica e da Saúde Hygeia* (2020): 193–201.

The Guardian. "Nature is Taking Back Venice: Wildlife Returns to Tourist-free City." March 20, 2020. https://www.theguardian.com/environment/2020/mar/20/nature-is -taking-back-venice-wildlife-returns-to-tourist-free-city

Universidade Federal de Juiz de Fora. "Pandemia e Meio Ambiente: Impactos momentâneos ou nova normalidade?" April 24, 2020. https://www2.ufjf.br/ noticias/2020/04/24/pandemia-e-meio-ambiente-impactos-momentaneos-ou-nova -normalidade/

Index

About the Contributors

Kátia Eilane Santos Avelar has a PhD in biological sciences and is Professor at Centro Universitário Augusto Mota, Rio de Janeiro. Her recent publications include the scenario of domestic violence in the first two years of pandemic.

Ricardo de la Fuente Ballesteros is a professor of Spanish literature at the University of Valladolid, Spain. He has numerous published articles and books. His current research includes culture and the environment. His recently co-authored book publication is *Mente, Cuerpo, Cultura y Educación* (2020).

Siddharth Singh Monteiro Bora has a master's degree in criminology and forensic sciences and is Associate Professor at Universidad de Ciências Empresariales Y Sociales, Argentina (Graduate Program in Forensic Sciences and Criminology). His field of interests are green crimes and vulnerable communities. Recent publications include *La Escuela Criminologica Ecologica y El análisis Factorial Multiplé: un studio de caso* (2020).

Zélia M. Bora has a PhD in Portuguese and Brazilian studies. Bora is on the Advisory Board to Ecocritical Theory and Practice, Lexington Books, and General Editor to Revista Interdisciplinar de Literatura e Ecocrítica. Bora's most recent publication is *Reading Cats and Dogs: Companion Animals in World Literature* (2021).

Marcus Alexandre Cavalcanti is engaged in a graduate program directed to local development. Cavalcanti has a PhD in education in health sciences at Federal University of Rio de Janeiro. The program has deep emphasis in the studies related to vulnerable communities. His recent article, "O Estado de Exceção nas Favelas: Perspectivas Biopoliticas a partir da Pandemia do COVID-19," represents this relationship.

Juan R. Coca is a professor at the Department of Sociology and Social Work, University of Valladolid, and director of Social Research Unit about Health and Rare Diseases. He is also director of book series "Biosocial World: Biosemiotics, and Biosociology." He has published in *Frontiers in Sociology*, *Biosystems*, and *F1000 Research*, among others. He recently co-authored a publication with Ricardo de la Fuente Ballesteros: *Mente, Cuerpo, Cultura y Educación* (2020).

Bruno Matos de Farias is a professor in the Program of Local Development at Santa Úrsula University. He is an architect and has focused his attention on civil constructions and sustainability. His recent book publication is *Engenharia na Prática: Construção e Inovação* (2022).

Georgina Vega Fregoso has a PhD in social sciences at the Centro de Investigaciones y Estudios Superiores en Antropología Social. She is a researcher from Conacyt Mexico. She also coordinates the master's degree in sociomedical sciences assigned to the Department of Social Sciences of the Centro Universitario de Ciencias de la Salud at the University of Guadalajara. Her most recent book publication is *Etnografía de la contamination. A Case Study in the Metropolitan Area of Guadalajara* (2022), edited by the University of Guadalajara.

Juan Pascual Gay is the author of different studies on Hispano-American and Spanish literature of the nineteenth and twentieth centuries. Among his titles are *El beso de la Quimera. A History of Decadence in Mexico (1893–1898)* (2012), and *El huésped del tiempo. Essay on Literary Ideas by Tomás Segovia*. His recent book publication is *El Clamor del Silencio. Ensayos sobre España, aparta de mí este cáliz* (2020).

María Fernanda Solórzano Granada is professor at the Intercultural University of Indigenous Nationalities "Amawtay Wasi." Her research is about socio-environmental conflicts, indigenous territoriality, and spiritualties. Among her most recent publications is "Espiritualidad en el airo (selva) un territorio insurgente en la nacionalidad siona del Ecuador."

Evely Vânia Libanori has a PhD in literature and theory of literature at Paraná State University, Maringá. Her field of research includes studies on alterity, human minorities, and humanities animal studies. She published several articles on Clarice Lispector and her relationship with animals. Evely is author of "Quem nos Habita" (2019).

Juarez Nogueira Lins is professor at State University of Paraiba. His field of research is mostly related to the Portuguese language and linguistics. His most recent co-edited publication is *Formação Docente e Experiências Didáticas* (2022).

Martha C. Galván-Mandujano is assistant professor of Spanish at California Polytechnic State University. Her research focuses on public memorialization in coordination with civil society organizations in Guatemala. She is currently working on the book *Nunca Más? Gendered Remembrance and Genocide Memorialization in Guatemala* co-authored (with JoAnn DiGeorgio-Lutz). Her co-authored chapter, "Gendered Remembrance, Collective Memory, Memorialization and Forgiveness: Cambodia and Guatemala," was published in 2020.

Maria Geralda de Miranda is professor in the Graduate Program at the University of Santa Úrsula, Rio de Janeiro, related to local development. The program has various projects on ecology, sustainability, and environment directed to the community. In the last two years, her articles were particularly directed to the impact of pandemics on vulnerable communities in Rio.

Animesh Roy is assistant professor at the Department of English, St. Xavier's College, Simdega (Ranchi University), in Jharkhand, India. His doctoral research was in the area of literature and postcolonial ecologies. His areas of research interest include environmental humanities, postcolonial studies, medical humanities, indigenous studies, gender studies, communication studies, and North-South discourses. His recent publications include *Provincializing Ecocriticism: Postcolonial Ecocritical Thoughts and Environmental-Historical Difference* (2021) and *From Clinical to Ecocultural: Literature, Health, and Ethnoecomedicine* (2022). His recent edited volume is titled *Ecology, Literature, and Culture: An Anthology of Recent Studies* (2022).

Norma Georgina Gutiérrez Serrano is a researcher enrolled in the Education Program of the Center for Multidisciplinary Research at National Autonomous University of Mexico since 1997. Serrano's most distinguished publication is *Espacios de Producción de Conocimiento en Educación en Mexiuco y el Cono Sur* (2014).

Mercedes Pascual Zavala studied a philosophy bachelor of arts degree at National Autonomous University of Mexico. Since 2018 she has been a part of the interdisciplinary research group Arte + Ciencia. Her fields of interest and work include melancholy, literature, sickness, and aesthetics. She has also collaborated on several literary projects.

Milton Keynes UK
Ingram Content Group UK Ltd.
UKHW011315240823
427424UK00006B/67

9 781793 654045